Ashtanga
YOGA
for beginners

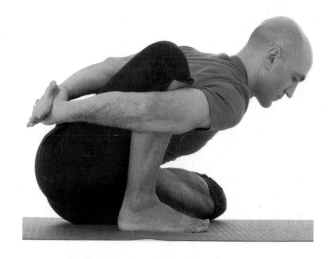

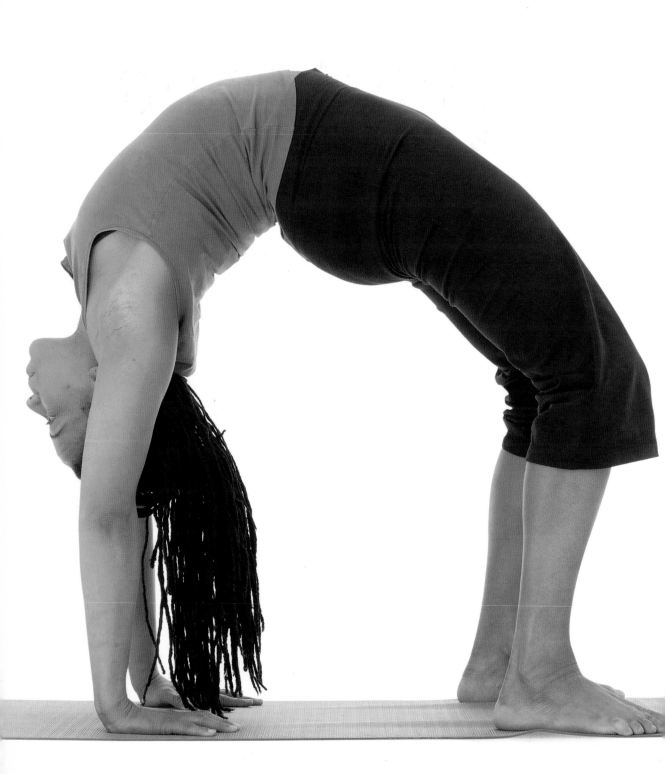

Ashtanga
YOGA
for beginners

Michaela Clarke

First published in Great Britain in 2006 by
Gaia Books, a division of Octopus Publishing Group Ltd
2–4 Heron Quays, London E14 4JP

Copyright © Octopus Publishing Group Ltd 2006

Distributed in the United States and Canada by
Sterling Publishing Co., Inc.
387 Park Avenue South, New York, NY 10016-8810

Michaela Clarke asserts the moral right to be identified as the author of
this work.

ISBN-13: 978-1-85675-270-1
ISBN-10: 1-85675-270-4

A CIP catalogue record for this book is available from the British Library

Printed and bound in China

10 9 8 7 6 5 4 3 2 1

Disclaimer
Any information given in this book is not intended to be taken as a
replacement for medical advice. Any person with a conditon requiring
medical attention should consult a qualified medical practitioner or
therapist before beginning any of the postures in this book. Whilst the
advice and information in this book is believed to be accurate and the advice,
instruction, or formulae have been devised to avoid strain, neither the
author nor the publisher will be responsible for any injury, losses, damages,
actions, proceedings, claims, demands, expenses and costs (including legal
costs or expenses) incurred or any way arising out of following the exercises
in this book.

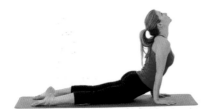
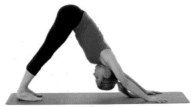
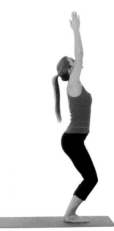

Contents

Introduction 6
Practising safely 8
Before you begin 10
How to use the course 12

Standing poses 14
Breathing, bhandas and dristi 16
Practising breathing and bandhas 18
Moving with the breath 20
Lesson 1 Sun Salutations 22
Lesson 2 Foundation Postures 46
Lesson 3 Standing Forward Bends 58
Lesson 4 Leg Balances 68
Lesson 5 Warrior Sequence 74

Sitting poses 82
Lesson 6 Sitting Basics 84
Lesson 7 Hip Rotators 92
Lesson 8 Bent-Knee Forward Bends 96
Lesson 9 Sage Postures 102
Lesson 10 Twisting and Boat Posture 108

Finishing poses 110
Lesson 11 Back Bending 112
Lesson 12 Beginning Inversions 116
Lesson 13 Shoulder Stand Sequence 120
Lesson 14 Head Stand Sequence 128
Lesson 15 Breathing and Relaxation 134

Quick reference chart 140
Index 142
Acknowledgements 144

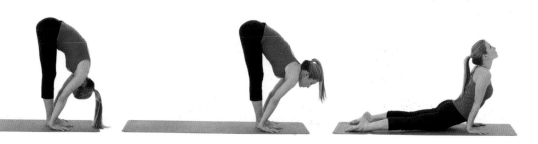

Introduction

Ashtanga Yoga has been increasing in popularity for several years, and has found its way into the press thanks to the many celebrities who enjoy this form of yoga. But it is not just a practice for celebrities, dancers and sports people. Ashtanga Yoga is a practice for anybody who wants to feel alive, happy, healthy, young, focused and full of light through every decade of life.

Many yoga pioneers became interested in yoga as children; others have visited India and practised regularly since they were teenagers. I admire and respect these people, and am deeply grateful for their courage and vision, but I'm not one of them. I will never forget the first time I was introduced to Ashtanga Yoga in 1989. Aged 24, I was working as a croupier in a casino. I smoked, drank a lot of alcohol and was utterly unenlightened and confused. The only philosophy I remembered was the French existentialism I'd learned at school, which claimed the only real choice we had as human beings was whether to commit suicide or not. I thought that was the truth. Somehow I found myself at the alternative holiday centre Atsitsa in Skyros, Greece, and it was there I witnessed Derek Ireland and Radha Warrell demonstrate the Primary Series. That beautiful demonstration sowed a seed that would, after several false starts, save and eventually radically change my life for the better. Seventeen years on, I feel happy; full of life, light and creative fire. I hope that for someone out there this book will have a similar effect.

I have been running Ashtanga Vinyasa Yoga courses for beginners for 10 years. I am often approached by people who have heard about the benefits of this wonderful practice and want to learn more, but don't have access to a teacher. Many excellent books describe Ashtanga Vinyasa Yoga, but until now none has broken down the sequence into easy-to-learn lessons and stages. Based on years of teaching experience, this beginner's course introduces the challenging yoga practice in a series of 15 lessons that allow you to build strength, flexibility and stamina according to your own ability and in your own time. Where necessary, I suggest alternative postures to allow you to work safely without straining. By the end of the course you will have a firm foundation in Ashtanga Vinyasa Yoga, and a practice you can take with you wherever you go.

What is Ashtanga Vinyasa Yoga?

A form of hatha yoga, Ashtanga Vinyasa Yoga was developed in Mysore, India, by Sri K Pattabhi Jois, known fondly to his students as 'Guruji'. It is based on ancient yoga traditions and relies on the practice of physical exercises to strengthen the body and still the mind in preparation for meditation. It is one of the most comprehensive exercise systems devised. Pattabhi Jois was 90 years old in 2005 (he seems to look younger every year), and still teaches students from all over the world in his new yoga centre in Gokalum near Mysore with his grandson, Sharath Rangaswami. He also undertakes a world tour every year.

Within the Ashtanga practice there are five increasingly difficult sets of postures. The first, known as the Primary Series, is the most important and is sufficiently challenging for most people. The lessons in this course are designed to help anyone learn the first half of the Primary Series. Pattabhi Jois is keen to point out that Ashtanga Vinyasa yoga is '99 per cent practice, one per cent theory.' This is an important lesson to remember. Talking, reading and thinking about yoga may be very enjoyable and interesting, but it's the work you do on the mat that gets results. Having said that, it is useful to understand something of the background.

The word *ashtanga* means 'eight limbs' and refers to the eight limbs of classical yoga, which were first described by the sage Patanjali some 2,000 years ago. No one is sure who Patanjali was – he may have been a doctor as well as a yogi – but he was one of the first people to put into writing teachings that had, until then, been ancient oral traditions passed down from guru to student. Patanjali wrote a series of aphorisms called the *Yoga Sutras* and in them explained in practical terms what yoga is, and how to use it to overcome the afflictions of the mind and reach a state of enlightenment. *Ashtanga* is used in the name of this form of yoga to indicate that all eight limbs should be considered when embarking on the practice.

The term *vinyasa* refers to the discipline of combining breath and movement. When one can seamlessly coordinate breath and movement, and keep the mind focused and clear, then the practice of yoga becomes a moving meditation. The set of more than 70 postures and linking movements that makes up the Primary Series should flow in time with the breath. Initially this practice may seem purely physical, but over time it can strengthen mind as well as body, healing emotional problems, with the ultimate intention of helping the soul evolve to its highest potential.

Who can do this practice?

Anyone with four limbs and a will to learn can practise Ashtanga Vinyasa Yoga. You don't have to be young and fit, you need only make a commitment to put in the time. If you have injuries or are ill, simply turn to the advice on pages 8–9 before beginning your practice. Then forget about being bad at sport, overweight, uncoordinated, unfocused or lazy. With Ashtanga Vinyasa Yoga you can and will change, as I did.

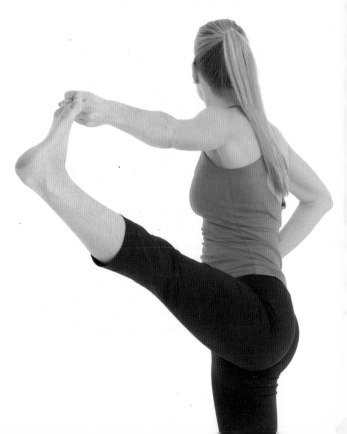

Practising safely

Ashtanga Yoga is a powerful form of bodywork and therapy, and there are a few common-sense rules to be aware of before you start to practise to avoid injury and maintain good health. There are also times when you should not practise.

Ashtanga Yoga has sometimes received bad press over the years, but it is a very safe practice as long as you follow the instructions in this book, work within your abilities, perform the postures in the correct order, and pay attention at all time. Most importantly, never throw or force yourself into postures. Instead work gently but firmly with the breath, keeping your limbs correctly aligned.

Menstruation
Women should not practise inversions during menstruation. Since Downward Dog is an inversion, this means no Ashtanga Yoga during the three heavy days of your period. Instead, use pillows to support your spine, bring your feet together and open your knees as pictured below.

Pregnancy
Although many advanced ashtangis practice, with modification, all through pregnancy and have perfectly healthy babies, it is not recommended that you begin learning Ashtanga Yoga while you are pregnant or trying to conceive. This form of yoga is a very cleansing practice that raises body temperature and massages the internal organs, and any kind of detox is a bad idea while you are pregnant. Wait for at least six weeks after having a baby and then begin to learn the practice gently, listening to your body and treating yourself with respect.

Illness
It's fine to practice if you have a cold, although it may be difficult to breathe at first (you may have to cheat and open your mouth). Ujjayi breathing and movement should help the nasal passages clear by the end of the Sun Salutations (see pages 22–45). Don't practise if you have a fever. Return to your practice when you are back in good health.

Injury
If you have a previous sports injury or imbalance, take the advice of a medical practitioner or sports therapist before starting this course, and proceed with extra care.

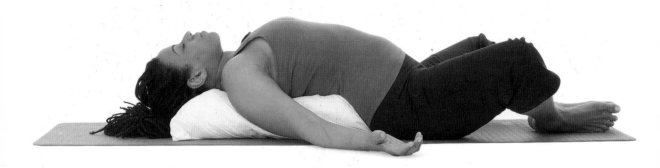

Common problem areas

If you experience pain while practising, be comforted that you are not alone. Some discomfort is normal for beginners to any form of challenging exercise. It's important to learn to distinguish between the beneficial ache of stretching and developing muscles (which eases if you breathe deeply) and pain in the joints, particularly the knees, which might indicate an old injury or a problem that needs medical attention. Described below are the most common areas of discomfort, with ways to minimize their effects:

Dizziness If you have low blood pressure, moving the head up and down and deep breathing may cause you to feel dizzy and faint. Try working more slowly until you get used to the movements. Yoga is best practised on an empty stomach, but some people with low blood sugar find they feel stronger if they eat something light to raise energy before a session.

Foot pain When working into Lotus Position, many students experience pain in the ankles and feet. This usually indicates that the foot is not high enough on the supporting thigh, which puts strain on the ankle. Use the modifications suggested in relevant poses.

Knee pain Knees are a common point of weakness for those who practise many sports, not just yoga. If you have stiff hips, you may put too much pressure on the knees in Lotus Position and other knee-bending postures. You might like to see a sports-injury specialist or physiotherapist for advice on how to open the hips without putting strain on the knees. Modify your routine until the pain goes away or practise under the supervision of an experienced teacher.

Hamstring injury If you follow the Sun Salutations and Vinyasas and work into forward bends with the breath, it is highly unlikely that you will suffer hamstring injury. If you already have an injured muscle at the back of the leg, gentle stretching may speed up healing

Lower back pain Yoga has been shown to be the number one cure for back pain, but make sure you don't add to the problem with incorrect posture. Take care to emphasize the bandhas (see pages 17–21), and if you are weak in the arms, don't let the pelvis slump to the floor in Sun Salutations and Vinyasas; instead use the modification with knees on the floor. Always be aware in back bends that the entire spine must arch to avoid putting too much pressure on the lower back.

Neck and shoulder pain Hunching the shoulders during Sun Salutations, Vinyasas and forward bends can lead to a cricked neck and stiff shoulders. Remember to release your shoulders down and back throughout your practice and when you feel tense take time out for a back rub.

Weak wrists If your wrists are weak, you may experience sudden, sharp pain when putting your weight into your hands. This is relatively common in people whose work requires repetitive movements of the hands. I suffered myself after several years as a sculptor. Create space in the wrists by standing on the palm of the hand and pulling up to stretch the wrist. You can also work in poses with fingers together rather than spread, or, if necessary, come up onto your fists for as long as is necessary. As your wrists slowly strengthen, the pain will lessen.

Before you begin

The one thing you must do before starting Ashtanga Yoga is to buy a sticky mat, available in a myriad colours in sports and health stores and on the Internet. You might look for one with a hessian weave that prevents the mat becoming slippery – a big advantage for beginners. Don't try practising on an old-fashioned foam hatha yoga mat – it doesn't work.

Most people get sweaty during practice: you might like to place a washable cotton yoga mat over your sticky mat. This is not only hygienic, it extends the life of your rubber mat. Spray the top and the bottom of the cotton mat with water before you begin practising to prevent your hands and feet from slipping.

What to wear

If you are following the course at home on your own, don't worry too much about what to wear as long as it's comfortable and easy to move in. You could practise in your underwear or pyjamas if you prefer. When practising with other people there are issues to be aware of. Take a shower before a communal class: natural body odours become more pronounced with the release of toxins during yoga practice, particularly in beginners. Then make sure your clothes cover your breasts, buttocks and genitals completely and at all angles, particularly when you are bending over: popping-out body parts distract you and other yogis. I find stretchy cotton lycra clothing best to work in. Baggy clothes can get in the way.

When to practise

If you can, practise in the morning on an empty stomach. Don't drink during, or for 15 minutes before and after, the practice. Use the

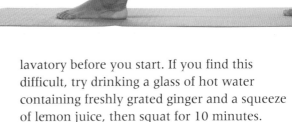

lavatory before you start. If you find this difficult, try drinking a glass of hot water containing freshly grated ginger and a squeeze of lemon juice, then squat for 10 minutes.

Traditionally, Ashtanga Yoga is practised six days a week with time off on Saturdays, and at the full moon and new moon. I strongly encourage you to follow this schedule, but if this is not possible, I suggest you practise each stage of the course (see pages 12–13) at least six times, taking no more than two days off between, before moving on to the next stage. You can take longer if you wish: since this is a practice that can last a lifetime, there's no need to hurry.

Where to practise

You don't need to set aside a special room for yoga. Any space large enough for you to spread out your mat and lift your arms straight up and out to the sides will do. Some people move a coffee table and practise in the sitting room; others find a space at the end of the bed. I even know of one yogi who spent years practising in his mother's bathroom.

Practice partners

Although yoga is a process of self-exploration, it can be helpful to begin with someone else. You might like to team up with a friend or even a group of people to work through the lessons in the book. This has several advantages. When you work with others, you are far more likely to stick to your target rather than be distracted by a floor that needs vacuuming or a sudden feeling of tiredness. Secondly, it is sometimes difficult to know whether you are doing the postures correctly unless you work in front of a large mirror, and I don't recommend practising more than once or twice in front of a mirror – it's too distracting. Having a friend check your posture from time to time can be helpful, but don't let others manipulate you unless they know what they're doing. Finally, if you team up with a friend you can read out the lessons for each other, which is almost as good as having a teacher.

You should make sure that you team up with someone who takes the practice seriously; save the socializing for after yoga sessions. I remember asking Pattabhi Jois's grandson, Sharath, about the Indian ladies' classes being taught in the afternoon. He told me they were '99 per cent chatting, one per cent practice'. Not ideal!

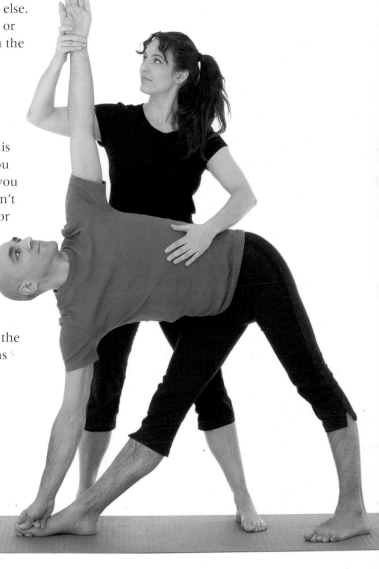

How to use the course

When a student learns Ashtanga Yoga in Mysore, India, his or her ability to memorize the sequence is considered as important as the ability to get into postures. One might spend several weeks simply learning the basics and Sun Salutations. No one ever goes beyond what they can remember, nor practises postures out of sequence. There is much to be said for this approach. It allows each student to work safely at his or her own pace. It forces students to pay attention, teaches them to focus, and, moreover, prevents a student from becoming dependent on the teacher.

The rules of the course

• Practise each stage of the course for at least six days (and longer if desired) before moving to the next stage.

• Do not skip postures or alter the order of postures.

• Do take one day off a week.

• Practise with care or not at all on full or new moon days.

• Don't take more than two days off per week (unless you are menstruating).

• When you don't have much time, set aside 10–15 minutes to practise a few Sun Salutations followed by the breathing and relaxation sequences.

In this book I encourage you to follow the system taught in Mysore. In other words, you need to memorize all the moves in one lesson before moving on to the next lesson. In this way you gradually build up your practice until, by the time you have finished the book, you have a firm foundation in the Primary Series. This book deviates slightly from the teaching in Mysore in that I suggest alternatives to some postures that I have found to be of benefit to my students.

Following the routine

In order to get the most out of the book and this beautiful form, it is important to stick to the order given. Each posture is presented to open and prepare the body for those that follow, so please don't skip lessons or try postures before you're ready. Be patient! As Pattabhi Jois says, 'Practice, practice, practice, all is coming...'. If you're tired, or do not have sufficient time to complete all the lessons you have learned, just practise the Sun Salutations from Lesson 1, followed by the breathing and relaxation in Lesson 15. Practising a little regularly is much better for you than doing nothing for a week and then attempting the whole book. Modify the lesson plans suggested at the start of each chapter to fit in with your own needs, but try to keep to the rules set out here.

LESSON 1

The lessons open with an introduction to the foundation of the practice. How to breathe, how to hold the *bandhas*, or body locks, and the principles of *dristi*, or gaze. In addition, there are the Sun Salutations that begin every practice session.

LESSONS 2–5

These sequences introduce standing and balancing postures, very important warm-up poses that prepare you for the deeper stretches to come. This sequence, and all subsequent sequences, must be practised in the correct order. That means you always practise Lesson 1 before going on to Lesson 2. When you have memorized Lesson 2, you practise Lessons 1 and 2 before going on to Lesson 3, and so on. In this way your practice lengthens and becomes more complex week by week, allowing you to build strength, stamina and flexibility gradually. The memorizing also improves your focus and ability to still the mind.

LESSONS 6–10

Once you have learned the Sun Salutations and standing postures, you are ready to tackle the Primary Series itself. This series of seated postures is known as *yoga chikitsa*, or yoga therapy. It continues and deepens the benefits of the standing postures, realigning, strengthening and toning the body while

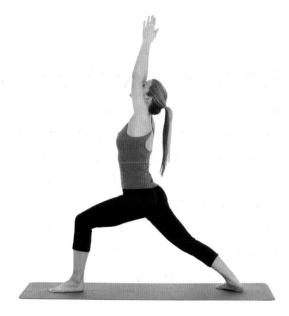

stilling the mind. If you would like to lengthen your yoga sessions, you can practise the Vinyasas (linking movements) before swapping sides as well as between postures. This increases stamina.

LESSONS 11–15

The finishing postures include inversions and so should not be practised by menstruating women, nor by anyone with a neck injury. On the other hand, practised correctly and at the right time, these are wonderfully invigorating and rejuvenating postures, which test and develop both physical and mental courage and balance. Finally comes a breathing sequence and relaxation exercise that is used to end all the lessons. The ability to relax after making effort is very important and you should never be tempted to leave out this stage.

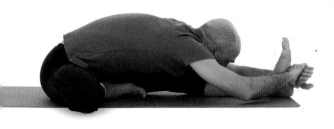

Standing poses

Take a little time before beginning Lesson 1 to practise the breathing and body locks demonstrated on pages 16–21.
Once you can make a smooth noise with your breathing and understand the body locks you are ready to start your first lesson proper. You may want to spend a few weeks working on the lessons you have already learned, improving your stamina and flexibility, and making sure you know the order of the postures. When you can practise stage five in about 45 minutes without referring to the book, you are ready to move to the sitting poses in the next chapter.

Lesson plan

First day
Learning the basics (see pages 16–21)
Lesson 1 (see pages 22–45)
Lesson 15 (see pages 134–39)

Stage one
Lesson 1 (see pages 22–45)
Lesson 15 (see pages 134–39)

Stage two
Lesson 1 (see pages 22–45)
Lesson 2 (see pages 46–57)
Lesson 15 (see pages 134–39)

Stage three
Lesson 1 (see pages 22–45)
Lesson 2 (see pages 46–57)
Lesson 3 (see pages 58–67)
Lesson 15 (see pages 134–39)

Stage four
Lesson 1 (see pages 22–45)
Lesson 2 (see pages 46–57)
Lesson 3 (see pages 58–67)
Lesson 4 (see pages 68–73)
Lesson 15 (see pages 134–39)

Stage five
Lesson 1 (see pages 22–45)
Lesson 2 (see pages 46–57)
Lesson 3 (see pages 58–67)
Lesson 4 (see pages 68–73)
Lesson 5 (see pages 74–81)
Lesson 15 (see pages 134–39)

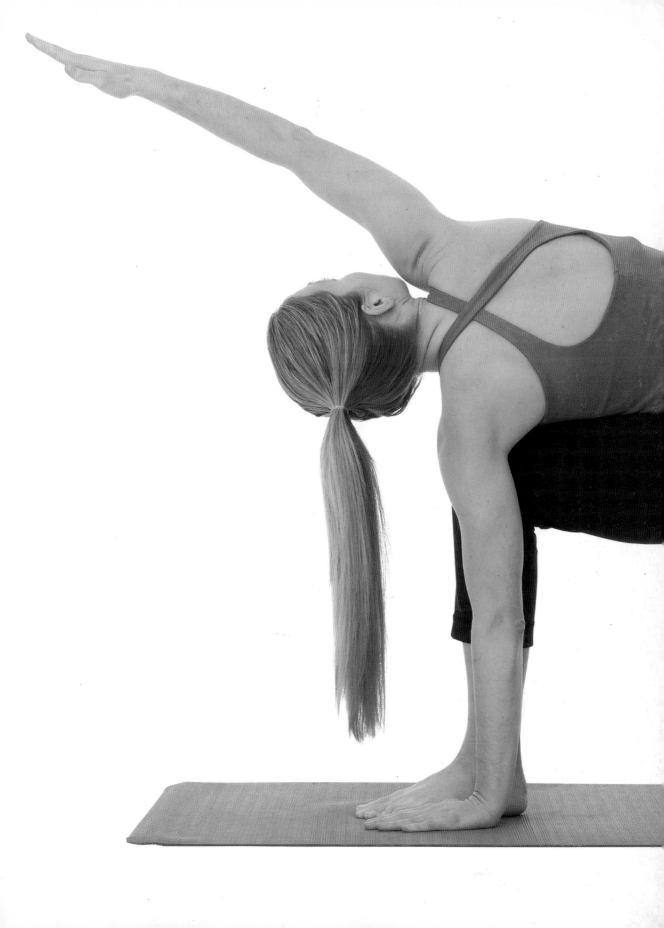

Breathing, bandhas and dristi

Once you have decided what to wear and where to practise, roll out your mat and sit down with the book. First read pages 16–21, then practise the exercises on breathing (see page 18), bandhas (see page 19) and moving with the breath (see pages 20–21) before moving on to Lesson 1.

Breathing

Throughout the practice you use a 'voiced' breathing style called Ujjayi breathing. Ujjayi means 'victorious', and this breath is designed to help overcome physical and emotional obstacles. You make the distinctive sibilant Ujjayi breath sound by gently contracting the muscles at the back of the throat.

There are several reasons for contracting the throat in this way. Firstly, being able to hear the breath emphasizes its importance while you move through the postures. This helps keep the mind focused. Secondly, it relieves pressure in the nasal passages, preventing them from blocking up and allowing a free flow of air to the lungs. This is particularly important for beginners who may get slightly out of breath during Sun Salutations. Maintaining pressure in the throat also allows breath to be drawn in evenly through both nostrils. In addition, air is heated slightly on the inhalation, helping increase body temperature, which, in turn, improves flexibility.

Breath is connected to and expresses moods and emotions. When we are excited or scared, breathing becomes shallow and quick; when we are calm we breathe deeply and smoothly. If you can learn to control your breathing you are also able to control your state of mind. When practising the postures of the Ashtanga Vinyasa sequence, allow the sound of your breath to consciously calm and focus your mind.

Linking movements with breath

In Ashtanga Yoga, breathing is continuous and rhythmic, an unbroken chain of inhalation and exhalation that links movements and measures the time you spend in each posture. The process of linking breath and movement is known as Vinyasa. Starting each step of the postures in the book you will find a breath instruction, which you should try to follow. Someone who has been practising this form of yoga for some time will not usually need to take extra breaths while going into and coming out of the postures. But even the most experienced student needs to take extra breaths from time to time when working into difficult or new positions and it is much better to take extra breaths than to hold the breath or rush into postures incorrectly.

It is possible to take extra breaths without interrupting the flow of your practice if you observe some basic principles of breath and movement. As a rule, lifts, extensions, opening or upward movements and back bends are performed on an inhalation.

Whereas downward, backward, folding, twisting or contracting movements are performed on an exhalation. For example, you inhale to extend your spine and exhale to fold forward. The key to taking extra breaths during practice is to take them consciously, match them to an appropriate movement and to keep them the same length as the rest of your breathing.

Body locks

The term bandha means 'lock' or 'seal'. In this context it denotes a muscular contraction at specific points in the body throughout the practice. In the Primary Series, two bandhas are used: Mula Bandha and Uddiyana Bandha.

Mula Bandha or 'root lock' is achieved by contracting the anal sphincter muscles. Women may find it helpful to contract the cervix, too. Mula Bandha requires a great deal of concentration and is emphasized while jumping, since its upward direction of energy helps you 'fly'. Contracting this bandha during challenging postures helps relax the rest of the body and relieve pain.

Uddiyana Bandha means 'upward flying seal'. It is an inward and upward contraction of the lower abdomen, which remains lightly drawn in and still throughout the breath. When the abdominal muscles are contracted in this way they support and protect the lower back.

Drawing in the lower abdomen on the inhalation forces the lungs to expand out toward the ribs, rather than down into the abdomen, which helps increase lung capacity and cardiovascular fitness. The use of Uddiyana Bandha also encourages the diaphragm to massage internal organs, allowing fresh blood to circulate and improving the efficiency of the spleen, liver and digestive system.

The gaze

Dristi (pronounced 'drishti') means 'gaze point'. Various gaze points are used to encourage correct form in each posture and to maintain the concentration necessary to work toward a state of meditation. Those used in the Primary Series are as follows:

Nose *nasagrai* This dristi is used when standing in Neutral Position, in Upward Dog Posture to prevent overextension of the neck, and in other postures to avoid distraction. Beginners may find it painful to cross the eyes and look at the nose for a long time; looking along the nose to the floor is an alternative.

Thumbs *anjusta ma dyai* We usually look at the thumbs when extending the arms to emphasize the upward motion of the body, or, in the case of *Trikonasana*, to encourage the chest to open.

Third eye *broomadhya* This gaze, directed at the centre of the forehead, also encourages the upward and opening motion of the body and the lengthening of the spine.

Navel *nabi chakra* In Downward Dog Posture, we look at the navel by tucking the chin into the collar bone. This encourages the back to straighten rather than collapse downward, and assists in stilling the mind.

Upward *urdhva* Focusing the gaze upward is another opening dristi.

Hand *hastagrai* Gazing at the hand is advised to encourage correct alignment in *Parsvakonasana*.

Toes *padhayoragrai* It is important to look at the toes to lengthen the spine in forward bends.

Sideways *parsva* This gaze is used when balancing and in twists.

Practising breathing and bandhas

The best position in which to begin these exercises is sitting upright with legs crossed. If you cannot sit cross-legged, sit on a chair with your back straight and feet flat on the floor. Once you are sitting comfortably, close your mouth and breathe only through your nose. Adjust the timing of your breath so that the inhalation and the exhalation are the same length, with no pauses between breaths. In regular breathing, the exhalation tends to be longer, so you may need to speed the exhalation and slow the inhalation. This encourages deeper breathing.

Ujjayi breathing

1 Take 10 breaths. Practise keeping the inhalation and exhalation balanced.

2 Read this step aloud in a loud whisper. The muscles you use to whisper are the same you use in Ujjayi breathing. The difference is your mouth is shut and the whispering noise is contained within the breath.

3 Take a deep breath in and then, opening the mouth, contract the muscles at the back of the throat and whisper the noise 'Haaaa' as you exhale. Practise until the sound of the exhalation is smooth but easily audible.

4 Once you can make a satisfactory noise with the mouth open, close your mouth and repeat step 3, this time making the sound on both the inhalation and exhalation.

Take a minute or two to practise the breathing before moving on to the bandha exercises. Beginners often make strange noises or no noise at all, but with practice this breath can be mastered by anyone.

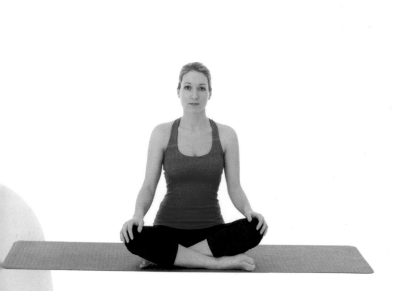

Floor posture

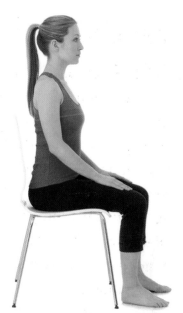

Chair posture

Mula Bandha

1 Continue Ujjayi breathing. Add in Mula Bandha by contracting the anal sphincter muscles at the end of each exhalation. Maintain the contraction as long as possible.

2 When you first practise, make the pressure fairly light, comparable to the wink of an eye. Wink one eye, then 'wink' the anus directly after to gauge the amount of contraction needed.

As your practice becomes more advanced and your pelvic floor muscles increase in strength, Mula Bandha should become more internal, particularly in women.

Uddiyana Bandha

1 Place one hand on your lower abdomen, between the navel and pubic bone. Place the other hand on your lower rib cage.

2 As you exhale, draw in the lower abdomen.

3 When you inhale keep the lower abdomen still. Let the area above the navel continue to move freely with the breath.

Spend a few minutes practising the breathing and the bandhas together before moving on.

Moving with the breath

Prop up your book on the wall in front of your mat. If you are working with a friend, one of you should read the instructions out loud, while the other partner performs the movements; then swap over. Later, practise together without using the book to memorize the moves. Begin by learning Ujjayi breathing, Mula Bandha and Uddiyana Bandha (see pages 18–19). Once you have established a rhythm to your breathing you may start to move.

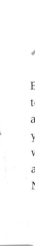

1 Stand facing forward with feet together (toe joints and ankle joints touching). Extend your spine, allowing your shoulders to open and relax down and back, and your arms to hang naturally by your side. Lift your toes, then your heels and shift your weight as necessary so you stand evenly on all parts of the feet. This is *Samasthitih*, Neutral Position.

2 **Inhale** Lift your arms out to the side, then above your head, bringing your palms together in Prayer Position. Tilt your head back and look up at your thumbs.

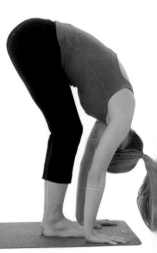

3 **Exhale** Bend your knees and fold forward from the hips, bringing your hands to the floor at shoulder distance apart. Pause here, breathing and checking your position. If you are flexible, your hands may reach to either side of your feet. If you are less flexible, take them further forward. Once your hands are on the floor, tuck in your head and let your weight come slightly back into your heels. Look at your nose.

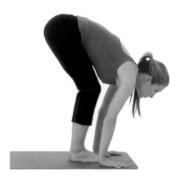

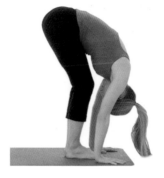

4 **Inhale** Bring your weight forward into the balls of your feet and the palms of your hands or fingertips. Draw back your shoulders, arch your back and look up.

5 **Exhale** Fold your head into your legs again and let your weight return into your heels. If you are flexible you may straighten your legs.

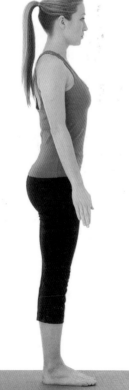

6 **Inhale** Come back up to standing, bringing your arms out to the side and over the head in Prayer Position again. Tilt your head and look up at your thumbs.

7 **Exhale** Bring your arms down to your side and your head facing forward. Practise this set of postures 10–20 times until you find it easy to coordinate breath and movement. When you are ready you can move to Lesson 1.

Sun Salutation A

Surya Namaskara A The Sun Salutation is a series of movements designed to still the mind and warm the body. In order to stretch safely later on in the practice it helps to be hot, preferably sweating. Ashtanga Yoga teaches two forms of the sequence. Sun Salutation A comprises nine simple moves coordinated with the breath (Vinyasas) that stretch and strengthen the arms, legs and back. Sun Salutation B features 17 Vinyasas, and includes movements that begin to open the hips and shoulders, too. This is by far the most important and possibly the most difficult lesson in the book, so be patient with yourself and take all the time you need.

Preparation advice

Before attempting a complete Sun Salutation, try out the individual postures and linking movements to see which variations you prefer: the modified position or the full posture. It may take a while to get the hang of the flow. In the beginning, take as many extra breaths as you need between movements, but make sure you always follow the suggested breath for entering each posture.

The following pages demonstrate two variations of the Sun Salutations. The first (see pages 23–27) is a beginner's version with extra breaths and modifications to the postures. The second sequence (see pages 28–31) shows the full version to aim for with practice.

If you are unable to jump forward or backward into postures, begin by stepping or walking into position one foot at a time. When practising jumping, remember to activate the bandhas; your strength will build in time.

Benefits
Warms the body and strengthens the arms and legs. **Jumping** strengthens the knees and improves coordination and stamina. **Upward Dog Posture** stretches the spine, chest and quadriceps, while **Downward Dog Posture** stretches the calves and opens the shoulders.

Contraindications
Do not jump if you have knee or back injuries. If you have a prolapsed disc or sciatica, take medical advice before practising.

Modified sequence

1 Inhale Begin in Neutral Position at the front of the mat. Lift your arms out to the side and then above your head, bringing your palms together in Prayer Position. Tilt your head back and look at your thumbs.

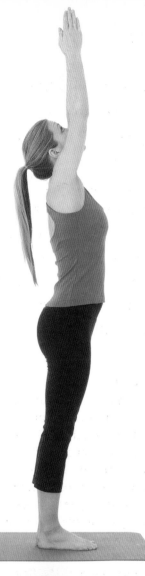

2 Exhale Fold forward from the hips. Bend your knees and bring your hands flat onto the front of the mat, shoulder distance apart. The less flexible you are, the more you will need to bend your knees and the further in front of the feet your hands will be. Tuck in your head and look at your nose.

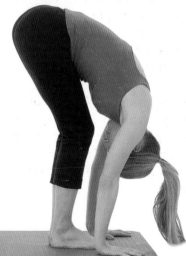

3 Inhale Arch your back and open your chest. To begin with you may not be able to keep your hands flat on the floor. Look up.

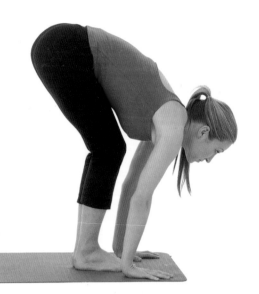

4 Exhale Step or jump your feet to the back of the mat, hip distance apart, coming into a push-up position. Lower your knees to the floor and bend your elbows to waist level. Look at your nose.

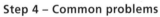

Step 4 – Common problems

Common problems in this position include hunching the shoulders, leading with the head, a saggy pelvis and elbows sticking out to the side.

If you are weak, start by working on the push-up position without bending your arms. Keep your shoulders open, lengthen your neck and pull your navel up toward your spine to support your back.

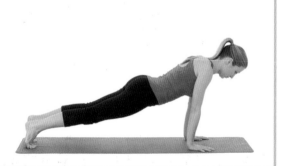

5 **Inhale** Push your chest forward, straighten your arms and roll over your toes to come into Upward Dog Posture. If you need to keep your knees and hips on the ground, bend your arms slightly so that you do not over-strain the lower back. Look at your nose.

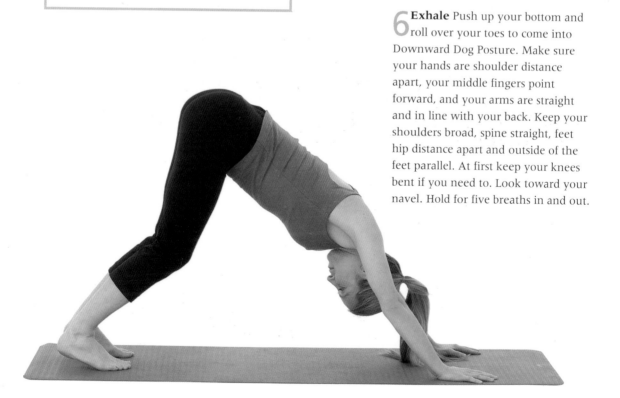

Step 5 – Rolling the toes

You will naturally roll over your toes if you keep your feet where they are and come into Upward Dog by pressing the chest forward.

6 **Exhale** Push up your bottom and roll over your toes to come into Downward Dog Posture. Make sure your hands are shoulder distance apart, your middle fingers point forward, and your arms are straight and in line with your back. Keep your shoulders broad, spine straight, feet hip distance apart and outside of the feet parallel. At first keep your knees bent if you need to. Look toward your navel. Hold for five breaths in and out.

7 **Inhale** Walk, step or jump to the front of the mat, landing with your feet together in your starting position. Take care not to bounce into a squat if jumping forward. Look up.

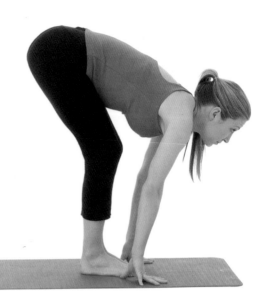

8 **Exhale** Forward bend toward your legs. Look at your nose.

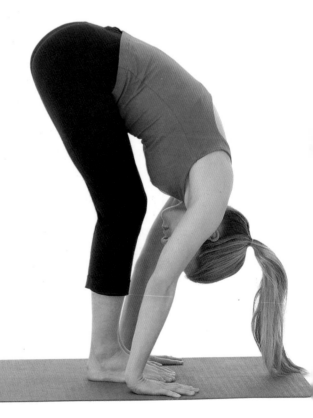

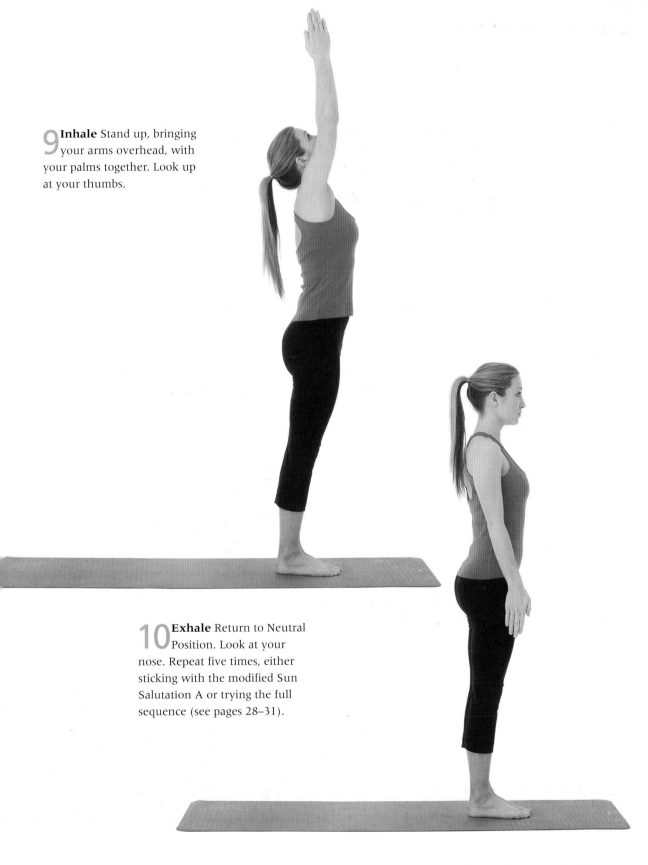

9 **Inhale** Stand up, bringing your arms overhead, with your palms together. Look up at your thumbs.

10 **Exhale** Return to Neutral Position. Look at your nose. Repeat five times, either sticking with the modified Sun Salutation A or trying the full sequence (see pages 28–31).

Full sequence

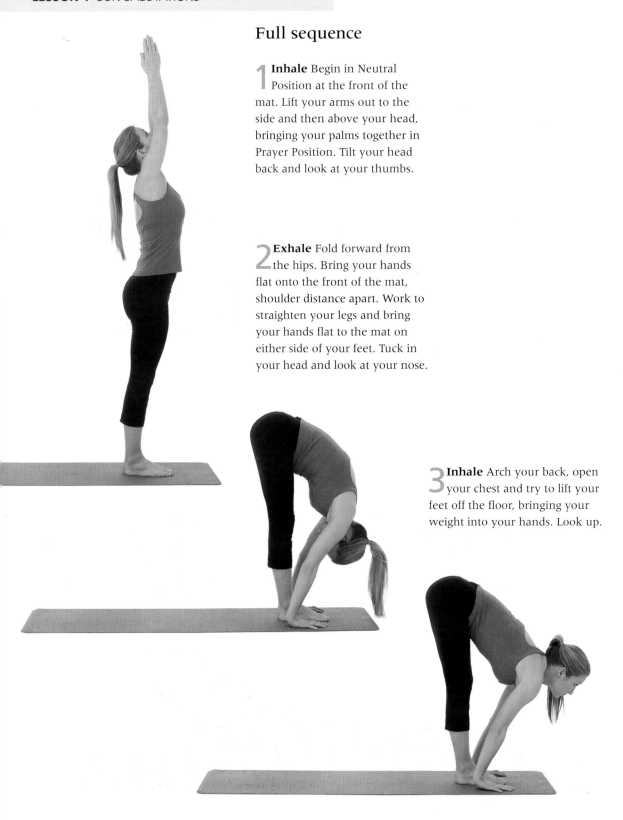

1 Inhale Begin in Neutral Position at the front of the mat. Lift your arms out to the side and then above your head, bringing your palms together in Prayer Position. Tilt your head back and look at your thumbs.

2 Exhale Fold forward from the hips. Bring your hands flat onto the front of the mat, shoulder distance apart. Work to straighten your legs and bring your hands flat to the mat on either side of your feet. Tuck in your head and look at your nose.

3 Inhale Arch your back, open your chest and try to lift your feet off the floor, bringing your weight into your hands. Look up.

4 **Exhale** Jump your feet to the back of the mat so that your feet are hip distance apart and you are in push-up position. From the push-up position bend your elbows and lower your body 5 cm (2 in) from the floor, keeping your chest, pelvis and knees off the mat. Look at your nose.

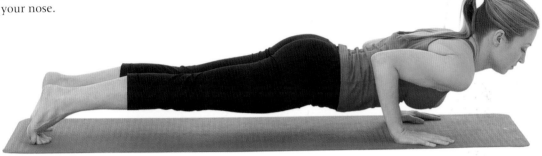

5 **Inhale** Straighten your arms, push your chest forward and roll over your toes to come into Upward Dog. Lift your knees and hips away from the floor and arch backward. Look at your nose.

6 **Exhale** Push up your bottom and roll over your toes to come into Downward Dog. Straighten your legs and press your heels to the floor. Look toward your navel. Hold for five breaths in and out. On the fifth exhalation, prepare to spring by activating Mula Bandha and bending the knees slightly.

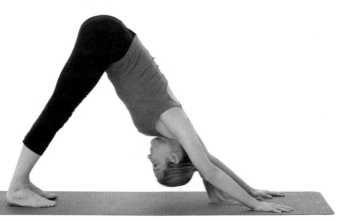

7 **Inhale** Jump to the front of the mat, landing with your feet together in your starting position. Keep your hands flat on the floor and your legs straight. Look up.

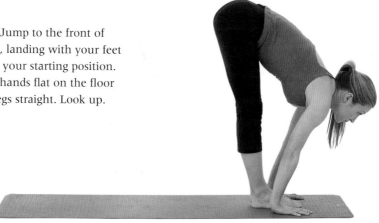

8 **Exhale** Forward bend toward your legs. Keep your legs straight while bringing your head toward your shins. Look at your nose.

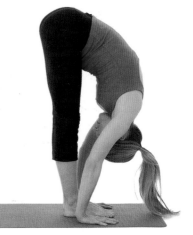

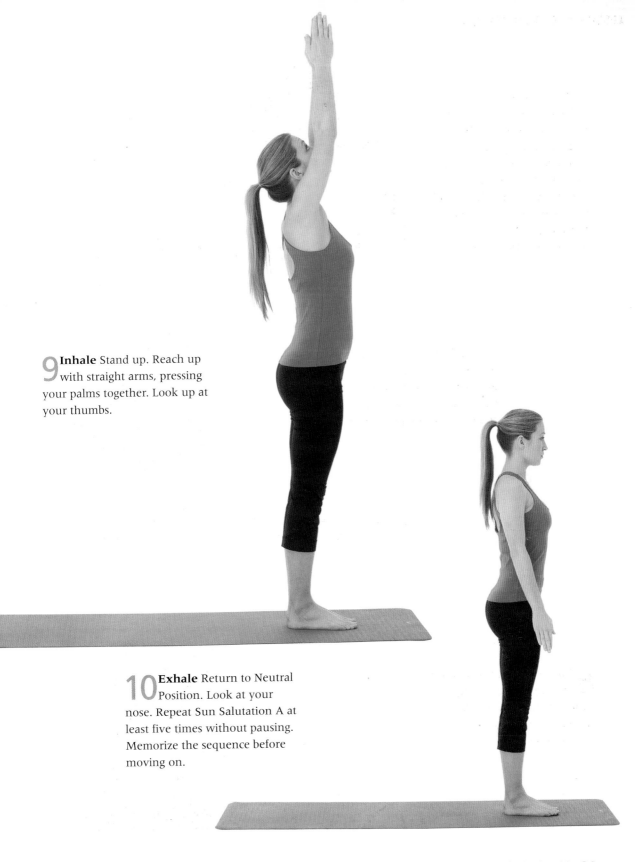

9 **Inhale** Stand up. Reach up with straight arms, pressing your palms together. Look up at your thumbs.

10 **Exhale** Return to Neutral Position. Look at your nose. Repeat Sun Salutation A at least five times without pausing. Memorize the sequence before moving on.

Sun Salutation B

Surya Namaskara B After completing five of these sequences, finish your practice by following the breathing and relaxation exercises in Lesson 15 (see pages 134–39).

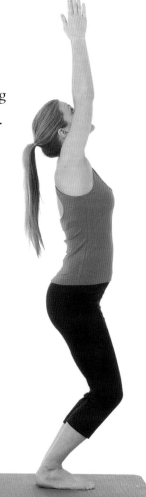

Benefits
Increases strength in the lower back, flexibility in the hips and shoulders, and overall endurance.

Contraindications
see Sun Salutation A, pages 22–31.

Modified sequence

1 Inhale Begin in Neutral Position at the front of the mat. Bend your knees deeply, keeping the heels down. Reach up with straight arms and bring your palms together. Look up at your thumbs.

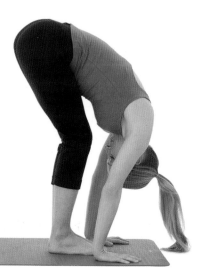

2 Exhale Fold forward from the hips, bending your knees if necessary, and bring your hands onto the front of the mat, shoulder distance apart. Tuck in your head and look at your nose.

3 **Inhale** Arch your back and open your chest. As a beginner, you may not be able to keep your hands flat. Look up.

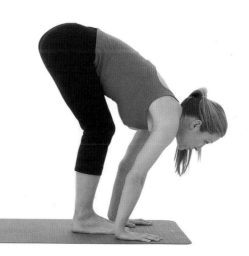

4 **Exhale** Step or jump your feet to the back of the mat, hip distance apart in a push-up position. Bring your knees to the floor and bend your elbows to waist level. Look at your nose.

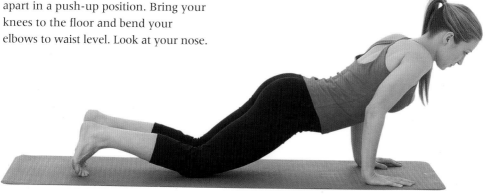

5 **Inhale** Push your chest forward, straighten your arms and roll over your toes to come into Upward Dog. If you need to keep your knees and hips on the ground, keep your arms slightly bent so that you do not over-strain the lower back. Look at your nose.

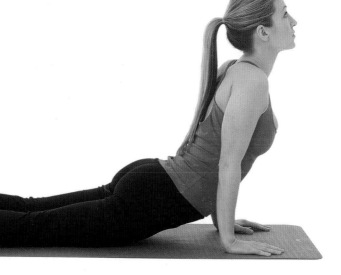

6 **Exhale** Push up your bottom and roll over your toes to come into Downward Dog.

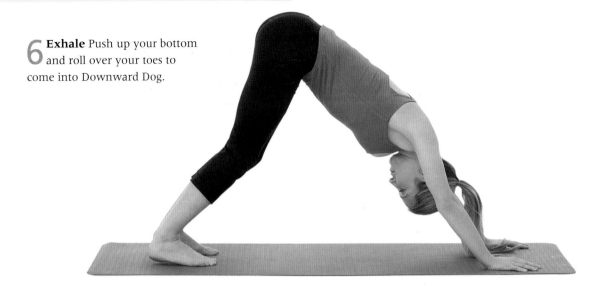

Step 7 – Stepping forward

If you find it difficult to step forward with your right leg, you just need to teach your body how to do it. Try the following manoeuvre, taking extra breaths where necessary: drop your left knee to the floor, step forward with your right foot, raise your left knee off the ground and turn your left heel in 45 degrees. You will then be in the position required for the next posture.

7 **Inhale** (extra breath) Step forward with your right foot.

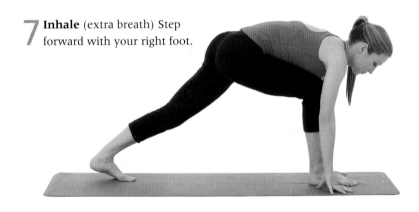

Exhale (extra breath) Turn your left heel in 45 degrees, keeping both heels aligned. Bend your front leg by 90 degrees so the knee is vertically above the ankle. Keep your left leg straight, foot well grounded. Make sure your hips and shoulders face forward.

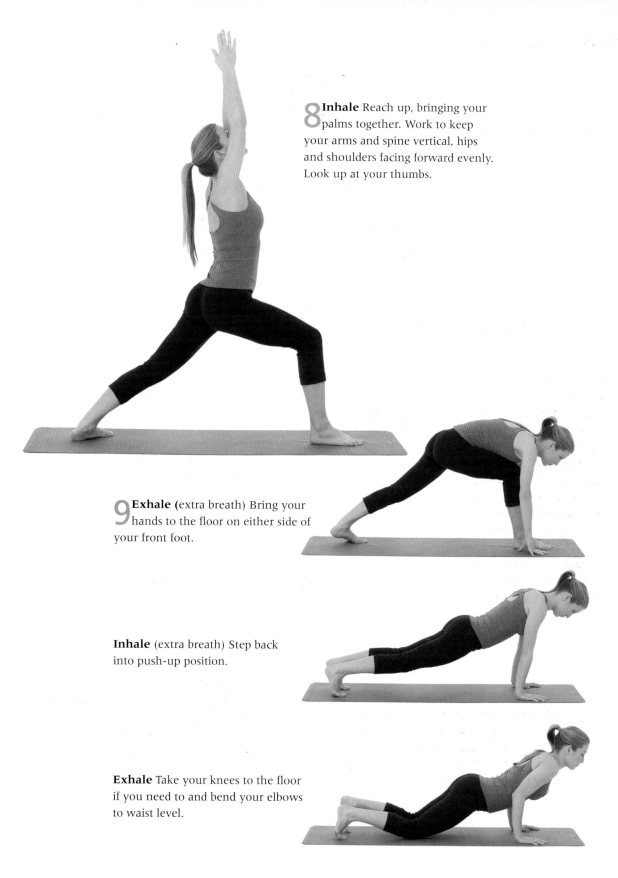

8 Inhale Reach up, bringing your palms together. Work to keep your arms and spine vertical, hips and shoulders facing forward evenly. Look up at your thumbs.

9 Exhale (extra breath) Bring your hands to the floor on either side of your front foot.

Inhale (extra breath) Step back into push-up position.

Exhale Take your knees to the floor if you need to and bend your elbows to waist level.

10 **Inhale** Push your chest forward, straighten your arms and roll over your toes into Upward Dog. If you need to keep your knees and hips on the ground, bend your arms slightly so that you do not over-strain the lower back. Look at your nose.

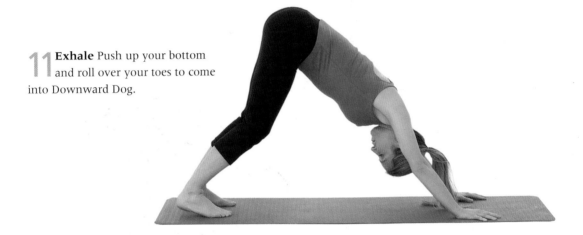

11 **Exhale** Push up your bottom and roll over your toes to come into Downward Dog.

12 **Inhale** (extra breath) Step forward with your left foot.

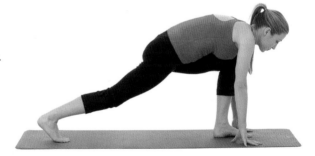

Exhale (extra breath) Turn your right heel in 45 degrees, keeping the heels in line. Bend your front leg by 90 degrees so the knee is vertically above the ankle. Keep the right leg straight and foot grounded. Make sure your hips and shoulders face forward.

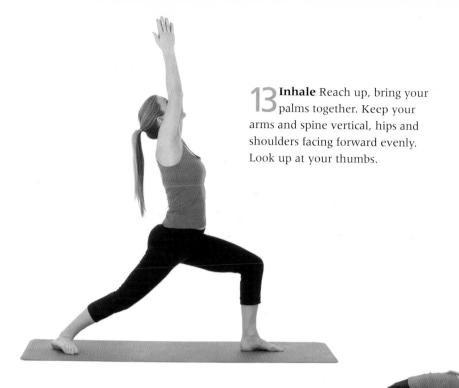

13 **Inhale** Reach up, bring your palms together. Keep your arms and spine vertical, hips and shoulders facing forward evenly. Look up at your thumbs.

14 **Exhale** (extra breath) Take your hands to the floor on either side of your front foot.

Inhale (extra breath) Step back into push-up position.

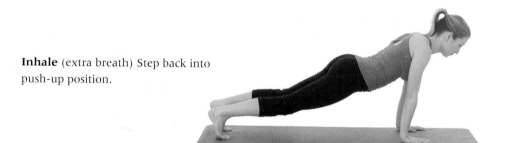

Exhale Take your knees to the floor if you need to and bend your elbows to waist level.

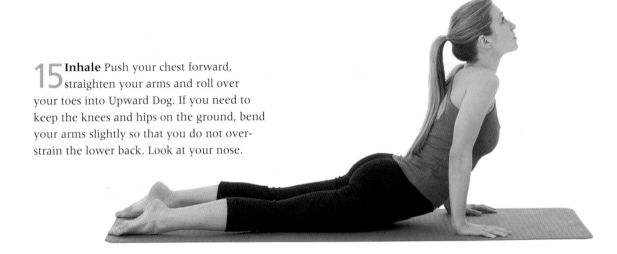

15 **Inhale** Push your chest forward, straighten your arms and roll over your toes into Upward Dog. If you need to keep the knees and hips on the ground, bend your arms slightly so that you do not over-strain the lower back. Look at your nose.

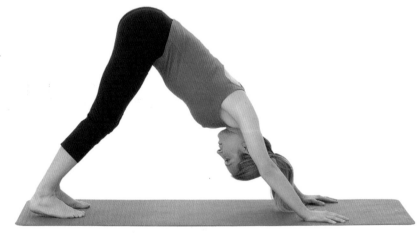

16 **Exhale** Push up your bottom and roll over your toes into Downward Dog. Look toward your navel. Hold for five breaths in and out.

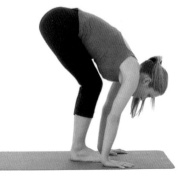

17 **Inhale** Walk, step or jump to the front of the mat, landing with feet together in your starting position. Take care not to bounce into a squat if jumping forward. Look up.

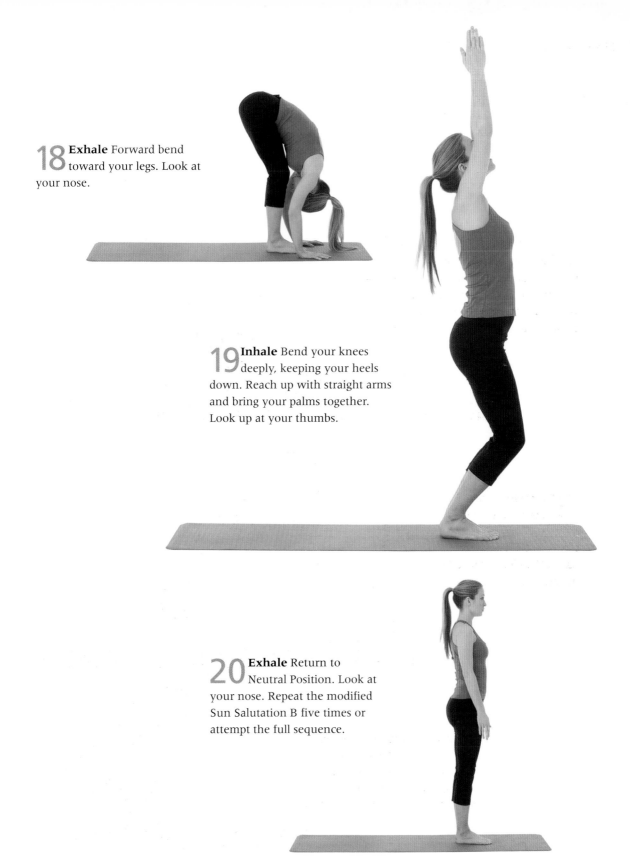

18 Exhale Forward bend toward your legs. Look at your nose.

19 Inhale Bend your knees deeply, keeping your heels down. Reach up with straight arms and bring your palms together. Look up at your thumbs.

20 Exhale Return to Neutral Position. Look at your nose. Repeat the modified Sun Salutation B five times or attempt the full sequence.

Full sequence

1 Inhale Begin in Neutral
Position at the front of the mat.
Bend your knees deeply, keeping
the heels down. Reach up with
straight arms and bring your
palms together. Look up at your
thumbs. If you have flexibility
within the ankles, aim for a
deeper squat.

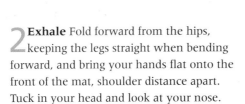

2 Exhale Fold forward from the hips,
keeping the legs straight when bending
forward, and bring your hands flat onto the
front of the mat, shoulder distance apart.
Tuck in your head and look at your nose.

3 Inhale Arch your back and
open the chest. Keep your
hands flat and lift your feet off
the floor, bringing the weight
into your hands. Look up.

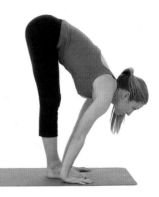

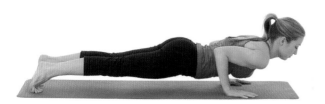

4 Exhale Step or jump your feet to the back of the mat, hip distance apart in a push-up position. Bend your elbows and lower your body to 5 cm (2 in) from the floor, keeping your chest, pelvis and knees raised from the mat.

5 Inhale Push your chest forward, straighten your arms and roll over your toes to come into Upward Dog. Lift your knees and hips away from the floor, and arch backward. Look at your nose.

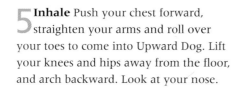

6 Exhale Push up your bottom and roll over your toes to come into Downward Dog. At the end of the exhale, turn your left heel in and step forward with your right foot.

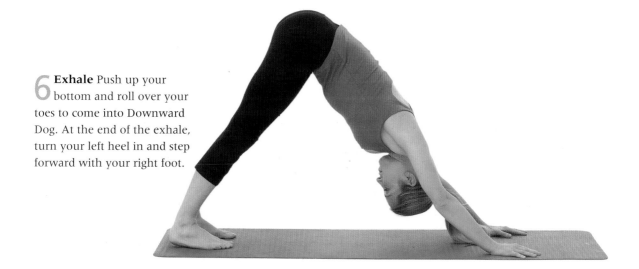

7 **Inhale** Reach up and bring your palms together. Look up at your thumbs.

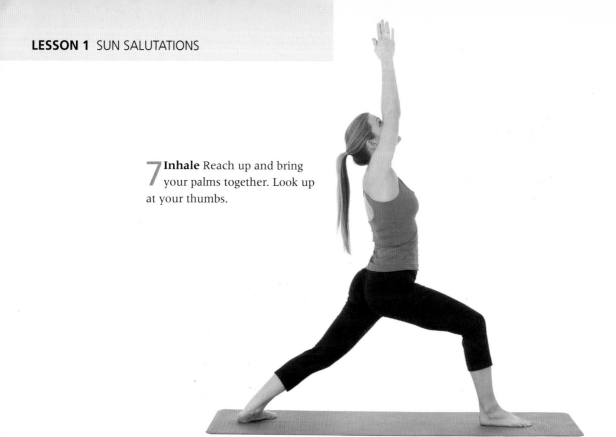

8 **Exhale** Bring your hands to the floor, step back into straight-legged push-up position. Bend your elbows and lower your body to 5cm (2 in) from the floor, keeping your chest, pelvis and knees raised from the mat. Look at your nose.

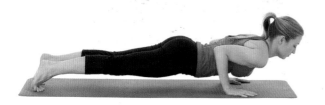

9 **Inhale** Push your chest forward, straighten your arms and roll over your toes into Upward Dog. Lift your knees and hips away from the floor, and arch backward. Look at your nose.

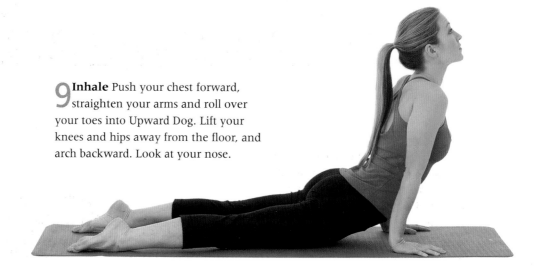

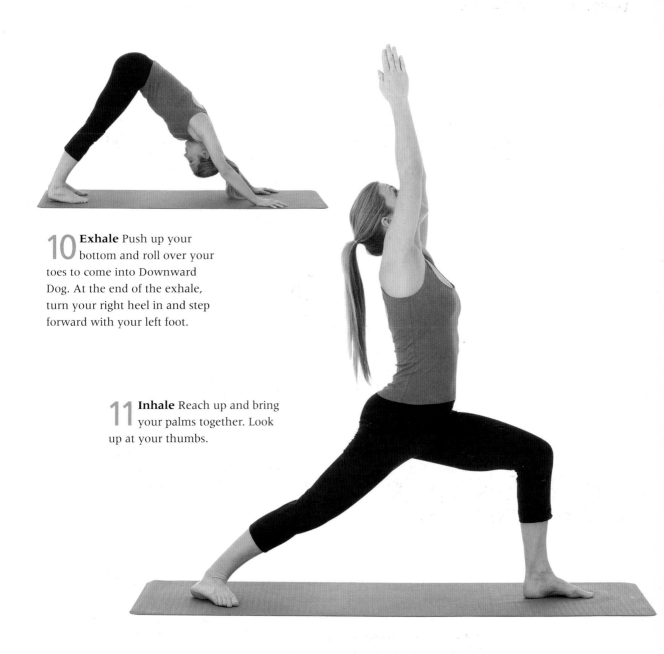

10 **Exhale** Push up your bottom and roll over your toes to come into Downward Dog. At the end of the exhale, turn your right heel in and step forward with your left foot.

11 **Inhale** Reach up and bring your palms together. Look up at your thumbs.

12 **Exhale** Bring your hands to the floor, step back into the straight-legged push-up position. Bend your elbows and lower your body 5 cm (2 in) from the floor, keeping your chest, pelvis and knees off the mat. Look at your nose.

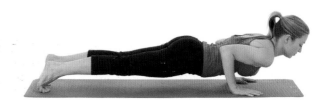

13 **Inhale** Push your chest forward, straighten your arms and roll over your toes into Upward Dog. Lift your knees and hips away from the floor, and arch backward. Look at your nose.

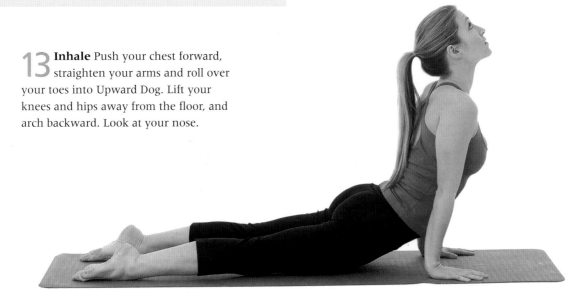

14 **Exhale** Push up your bottom and roll over your toes into Downward Dog. Look toward your navel. Straighten your legs and press your heels to the floor. Hold Downward Dog for five breaths in and out.

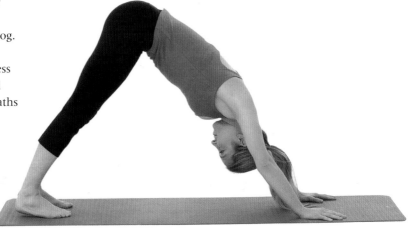

15 **Inhale** Jump to the front of the mat, landing with feet together in your starting position. Keep your hands flat on the floor and legs straight.

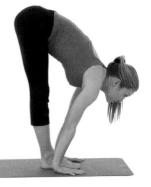

16 **Exhale** Forward bend toward your legs. Look at your nose. Work with straight legs, tucking your nose toward your knees.

17 **Inhale** Bend your knees as deeply as your ankles will allow, keeping your heels down. Reach up with straight arms and bring your palms together. Look up at your thumbs.

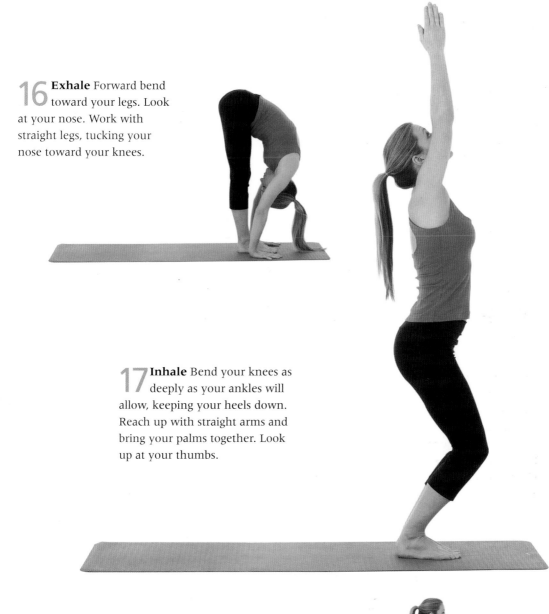

18 **Exhale** Return to Neutral Position. Look at your nose. Repeat Sun Salutation B five times.

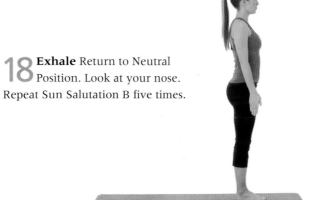

Bound Toe Forward Bend

Padangusthasana First, practise Lesson 1. You should be able to practise five each of Sun Salutations A and B, either modified or full variations, before proceeding.

Benefits

The forward bends, Triangle poses and side stretches in Lesson 2 help develop awareness of alignment and stretch and strengthen, while relieving tension throughout the body. They tone the waist and stimulate internal organs.

Contraindications

If you have a prolapsed disc or sciatica consult a physiotherapist or osteopath before practising yoga. If you are stiff, work into postures with knees bent.

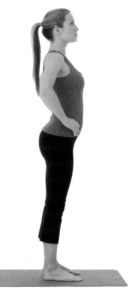

1 Inhale From Neutral Position, step or jump the feet shoulder distance apart, keeping the outside of the feet parallel. Place your hands on your waist and arch backward, still inhaling. Squeeze your fingers into your lower abdomen to assist you in drawing in and up on the Uddiyana Bandha.

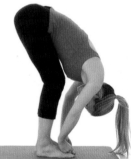

2 Exhale Fold forward from the hips. Bend your knees and grasp your big toes with your first two fingers and thumbs.

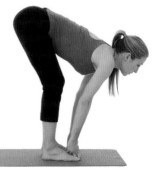

3 Inhale Keeping the grip on your toes, arch backward, drawing your shoulders back. Look up.

4 Exhale Fold forward and look at your nose. Hold the posture for five breaths in and out.

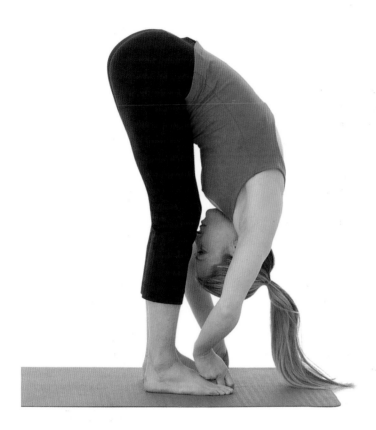

Step 4 – Stretching the legs

In every forward bend it is better to bend the knees to work into the posture before trying to straighten the legs. This helps release the muscles of the lower back. If your legs are straight, bring some of your weight into the balls of your feet. Lift your sitting bones to increase the stretch at the back of the legs.

Full posture

• Follow steps 1–4, but keep your legs straight.

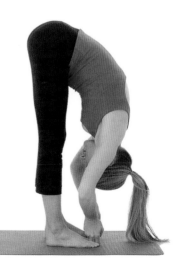

Hand to Foot Forward Bend

Padahastasana This is a continuation of the last posture; do not come out of the previous forward bend before starting this one.

1 Inhale Maintaining your grip on the toes from the previous posture, arch your back and draw your shoulders back as before. Look up.

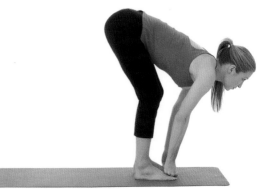

2 Exhale Fold forward again. Bend your knees if necessary. Take your hands, palms up, beneath the front of your feet until you are standing on the palms of your hands with your toes touching your wrists.

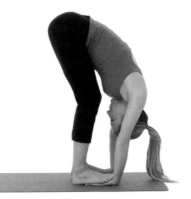

3 Inhale Arch your back and draw your shoulders back. Look up.

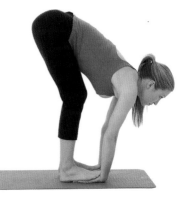

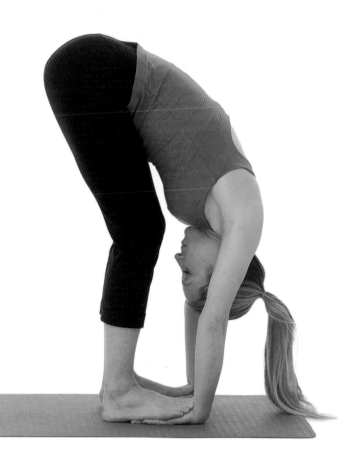

4 Exhale Fold in toward your legs, drawing your head down and bringing belly to thighs, chest to knees. Look at your nose. Hold the posture for five breaths in and out.

Full posture
• Follow steps 1–4, but keep your legs straight.

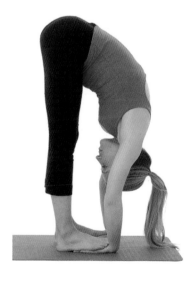

Coming out
• **Inhale** With hands still beneath your feet, look up.
• **Exhale** Bring your hands to your waist. Look at your nose.
• **Inhale** Come back up to standing.
• **Exhale** Step or jump back to Neutral Position.

Hand to foot forward bend **49**

Extended Triangle

Utthita Trikonasana Practise the same variation on both sides, even if you are more flexible on one side than the other. Pay particular attention to the alignment of your feet, as incorrect positioning can harm the knees and lower back. Work to keep the outside edges of the feet grounded and lift the arches.

Benefits

Reaching to the side teaches alignment and a sense of direction. This posture also stretches the waist, hips and shoulders.

Contraindications

See page 46.

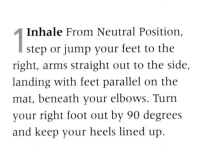

1 **Inhale** From Neutral Position, step or jump your feet to the right, arms straight out to the side, landing with feet parallel on the mat, beneath your elbows. Turn your right foot out by 90 degrees and keep your heels lined up.

Step 1 – Jumping into poses

At first, it is enough to step into postures from the front of your mat. When you feel ready, start to jump the feet into position, which helps strengthen the knee muscles. When jumping, start from the centre of the mat so both feet travel the same distance – yoga is all about balance.

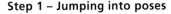

2 **Exhale** Fold to the right, looking down at your right foot. Bend your right knee until you are able to grasp your right big toe with the first two fingers and thumb of your right hand.

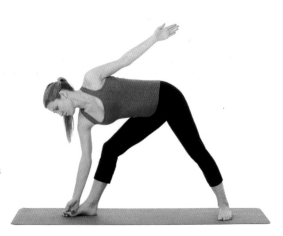

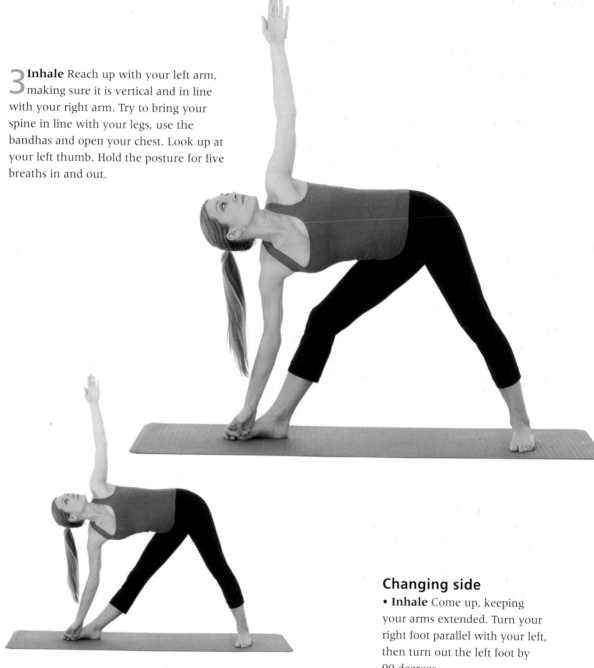

3 **Inhale** Reach up with your left arm, making sure it is vertical and in line with your right arm. Try to bring your spine in line with your legs, use the bandhas and open your chest. Look up at your left thumb. Hold the posture for five breaths in and out.

Full posture
• Follow steps 1–3, but keep your legs straight.

Changing side
• **Inhale** Come up, keeping your arms extended. Turn your right foot parallel with your left, then turn out the left foot by 90 degrees.
• **Exhale** Repeat the posture on your left side.

Moving on
• **Inhale** Come up from the left side and return your feet to parallel. Retain this foot position to move into the next posture.

Revolved Triangle

Parivrtta Trikonasana This is the first twist in the series. Keep the knees soft while working into all standing postures.

Benefits

Twists relieve backache, headaches, a stiff neck and shoulders. They improve spinal flexibility, open the hips and stimulate the digestion by massaging internal organs.

Contraindications

Do not twist after abdominal operations. Take medical advice if you have a hernia.

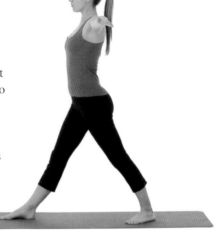

1 Inhale Starting from the wide-legged position of the previous posture, turn your right foot out by 90 degrees to point to the front of the mat. Turn your left foot in 45 degrees from the back edge of the mat. Turn your torso so your shoulders and hips face over your right leg. Keep your arms extended.

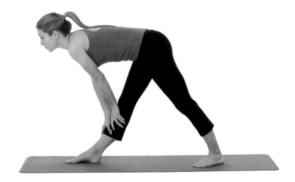

2 Exhale Fold forward over your right leg, sliding your hands down your right shin as far as they will go with your legs straight. Keep your hips even as you fold forward and keep your head in line with your spine. To go further into this position you must be flexible enough to bring your fingertips to the floor on either side of your foot.

Step 2 – Working with stiffness

If you are stiff and cannot bring your spine parallel with the floor, work on improving your forward bend before twisting. To do this, keep both hands on your front leg and focus on keeping your hips in line as you fold forward. Keep your head in line with your spine and hold this position throughout the posture. Do not twist.

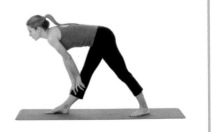

3 Inhale Keeping your left hand's fingertips on the floor inside your right foot, bring your right hand to your sacrum. Check that your hips are in line and your sacrum is parallel to the floor. Rotate your upper torso until your chest is open and flat. Look up. Hold the posture for five breaths in and out.

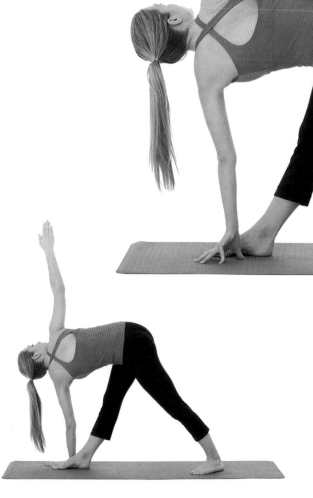

Changing side
• **Inhale** Come up to standing, keeping your arms extended. Turn your right foot out by 45 degrees and your left foot by 90 degrees.
• **Exhale** Repeat the posture on the left side.

Coming out
• **Inhale** Come up to standing with arms extended. Bring the feet back to parallel.
• **Exhale** Step or jump back to Neutral Position, facing the front of the mat.

Full posture
• Bring your left hand to the outside of your right foot and lift your right arm vertically to open your chest. Keep your spine horizontal and your arms vertical.

Side Stretch

Utthita Parsvakonasana I have added an extra breath to this intense hip and groin stretch to ensure that the chest and shoulders are positioned correctly. The full variation does not include the extra breath.

Benefits

Develops strength in the legs and flexibility in the upper back and shoulders.

Contraindications

See page 46.

---

1 **Inhale** Step or jump your feet to the right, extending your arms to the side. Land with feet parallel beneath your wrists. Turn your right foot out by 90 degrees. Keep your heels aligned.

2 **Exhale** Bend your right knee to bring it vertically in line with your ankle. Bend your right arm and rest your elbow on your right leg.

3 **Inhale** (extra breath) Reach up vertically with your left arm. Open your chest and bring your arms and shoulders into a vertical line.

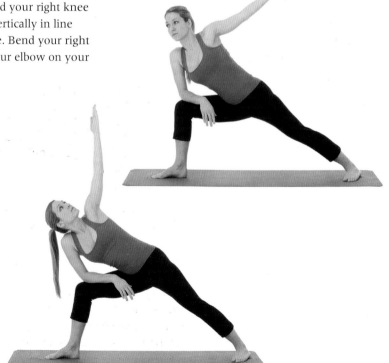

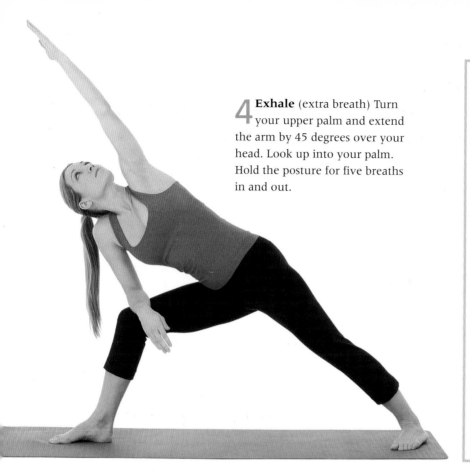

4 Exhale (extra breath) Turn your upper palm and extend the arm by 45 degrees over your head. Look up into your palm. Hold the posture for five breaths in and out.

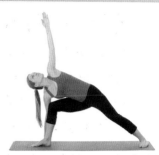

Step 4 – Stretching the arm

This is a side stretch; do not lean forward or arch the back in an attempt to take the arm to 45 degrees. Work instead on bringing your extended arm to vertical. If you wish to work toward the full posture, start by taking the fingertips of your lower hand to the floor on the outer side of your front foot.

Full posture
• Follow steps 1–3.
• **Exhale** Extend your left arm by 45 degrees over your head. Look up into your palm.

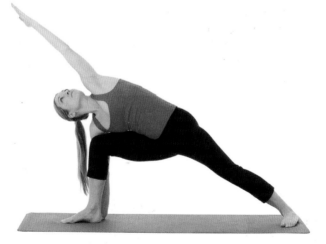

Changing side
• **Inhale** Come up to standing, keeping your arms extended. Change your feet so the left foot angles out by 90 degrees.
• **Exhale** Repeat the posture on the left.

Moving on
• **Inhale** Come up from the left side and return your feet to parallel. Retain this foot position as you move into the next posture.

Revolved Side Stretch

Parivrtta Parsvakonasana After completing this posture, finish Lesson 2 with the breathing and relaxation in Lesson 15 (see pages 134–39).

Benefits

Builds on the work of the previous postures and encourages the lungs to expand.

Contraindications

Do not twist after abdominal operations. Take medical advice if you have a hernia.

1 Inhale Maintaining the wide-legged position from the previous posture, turn your right foot out 90 degrees to point to the front of the mat. Turn your left foot in 45 degrees from the back edge of the mat. Turn your entire torso so your shoulders and hips face over your right leg.

2 Exhale Bend your right knee to 90 degrees and bring your back knee to the floor. Twist and wedge your left arm behind your right knee. Work on bringing your left hand to the floor outside your right foot. Place your right hand on your lower back.

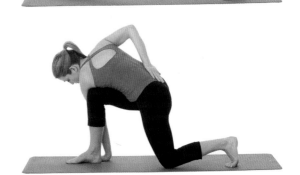

Step 2 – Working with stiffness

If you cannot bring your hand to the floor, try this variation with your hands in Prayer Position. These pictures show the position from the front and rear so that you can see exactly what to do.

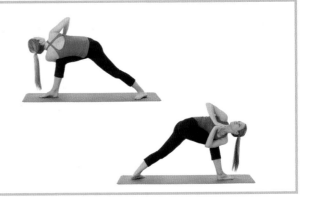

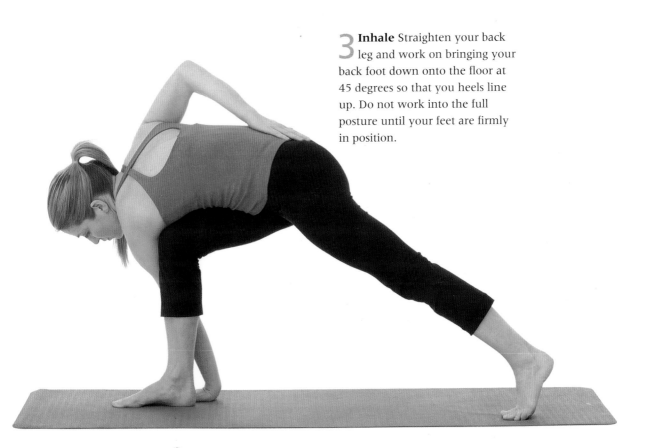

3 Inhale Straighten your back leg and work on bringing your back foot down onto the floor at 45 degrees so that you heels line up. Do not work into the full posture until your feet are firmly in position.

Full posture

• **Inhale** Once your feet are in position, reach up with your right arm, opening the chest and shoulders vertically, then bring the raised arm over your head at a 45-degree angle. Turn your palm to face the floor. Look up into your palm.

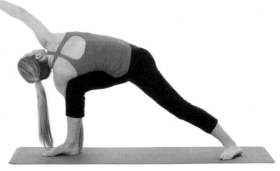

Changing side

• **Inhale** Come up to standing, keeping your arms extended. Change your feet so the left foot angles out by 90 degrees, your right foot by 45 degrees.
• **Exhale** Repeat the posture on the left.

Coming out

• **Inhale** Come up to standing with arms extended. Bring the feet back to parallel.
• **Exhale** Step or jump back to Neutral Position, facing the front of the mat.

Wide-legged Forward Bend A

Prasarita Padottanasana Before starting this lesson, practise Lessons 1 and 2 regularly until you know the sequence of postures by heart. Throughout this lesson be aware of your bandha control. Each time you bring your hands to your waist, press your fingers into your abdomen to encourage Uddiyana Bandha. Every time you exhale forward emphasize Mula Bandha.

Benefits

The forward bend continues to work on the flexibility of the back of the body and the shoulders. It also encourages bandha practice.

Contraindications

See page 46.

1 **Inhale** From Neutral Position, step or jump to the right, bring your legs 1–1.5 metres (3–4¹/₂ feet) apart with your feet parallel. Take your hands to your waist and draw back your shoulders and elbows to open the chest.

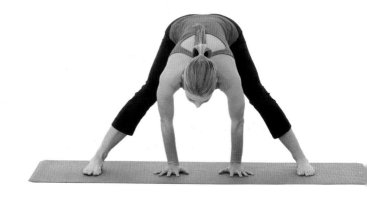

2 **Exhale** Bend your knees and fold forward, bringing your hands to the floor, shoulder distance apart. The position of your hands will vary according to your level of flexibility. Eventually they will rest between the feet; at first much further forward. Flatten your hands and keep your arms parallel.

3 Inhale Straighten your arms, arch your back, open your chest and look up.

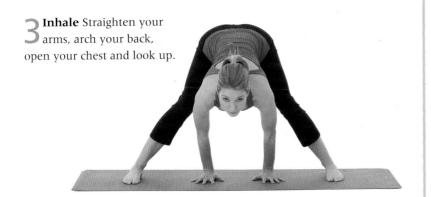

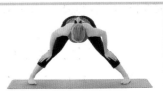

Step 3 – Working with stiffness

If you are stiff in the hamstrings and lower back, alternate a bent-knee variation of the posture to stretch the back with a straight-legged version to lengthen the hamstrings. Instead of bringing your hands to the floor, rest them on your shins.

4 Exhale Fold forward to bring your head toward the floor between your hands. Look at your nose. Hold the posture for five breaths in and out.

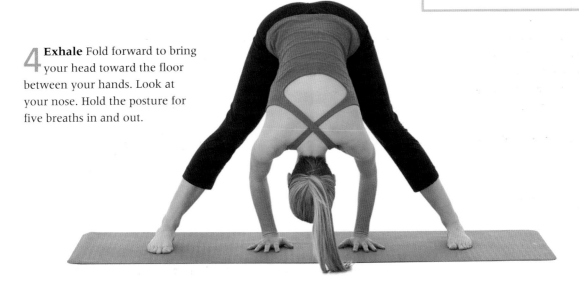

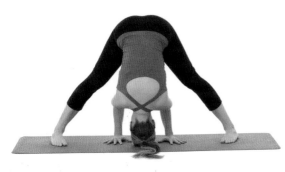

Full posture
• Follow steps 1–4, but take your head to the floor between your hands, keeping your legs straight.

Moving on
• **Inhale** Straighten your arms, open your chest and look up.
• **Exhale** Bring your hands to your waist.
• **Inhale** Come up to standing.
• **Exhale** Rest your hands on your thighs ready to start the next posture.

Wide-legged Forward Bend B

Prasarita Padottanasana Start this posture from the finishing position of the previous forward bend. Do not move the feet back to Neutral Position.

Benefits

The forward bend continues to work on the flexibility of the back of the body and the shoulders. It also encourages bandha practice.

Contraindications

See page 46.

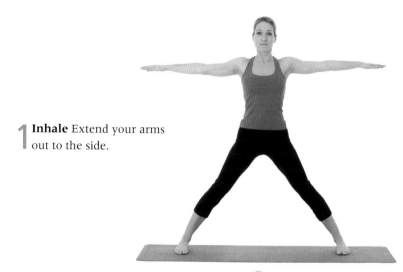

1 Inhale Extend your arms out to the side.

2 Exhale Take your hands to your waist.

3 Inhale Open your chest and shoulders.

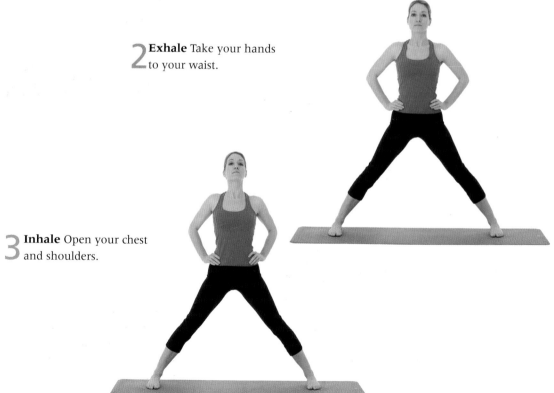

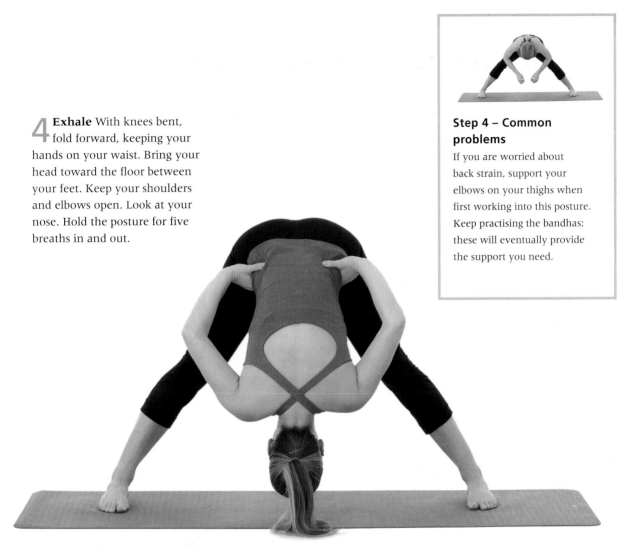

4 **Exhale** With knees bent, fold forward, keeping your hands on your waist. Bring your head toward the floor between your feet. Keep your shoulders and elbows open. Look at your nose. Hold the posture for five breaths in and out.

Step 4 – Common problems

If you are worried about back strain, support your elbows on your thighs when first working into this posture. Keep practising the bandhas: these will eventually provide the support you need.

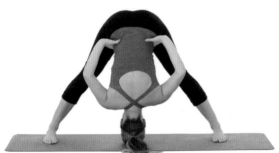

Full posture

• Follow steps 1–4, but keep your legs straight, extending your spine forward and taking your head to the floor between your feet.

Moving on

• **Inhale** Come up to standing.
• **Exhale** Rest your hands on your thighs ready to start the next posture.

Wide-legged forward bend B **61**

Wide-legged Forward Bend C

Prasarita Padottanasana If you cannot lace your hands
behind your back in step 2, start by holding opposite elbows
behind your back.

Benefits

The forward bend continues to
work on the flexibility of the
back of the body and the
shoulders. It also encourages
bandha practice.

Contraindications

See page 46.

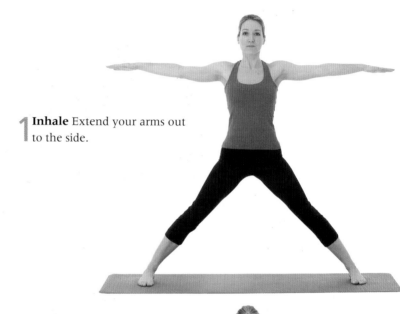

1 Inhale Extend your arms out
to the side.

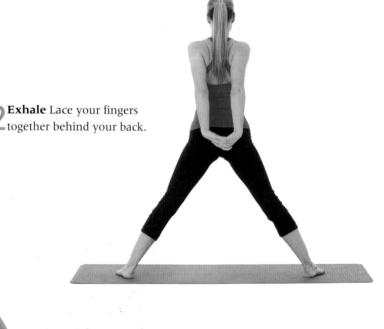

2 Exhale Lace your fingers
together behind your back.

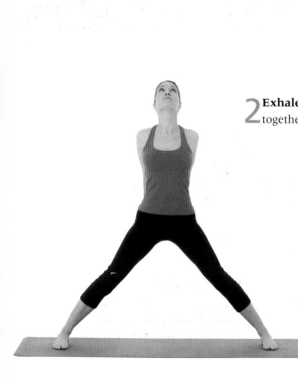

3 Inhale Straighten your arms,
opening your shoulders and chest.

4 **Exhale** Bend your knees and extend forward to bring your head toward the floor between your feet. Take your hands over the top of your head. Look at your nose. Hold the posture for five breaths in and out.

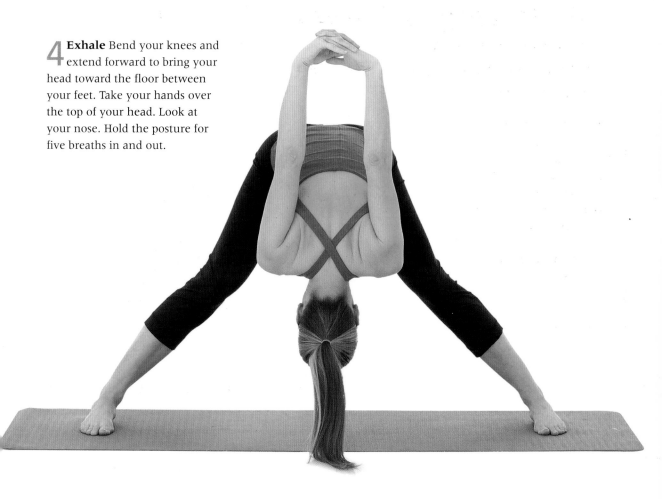

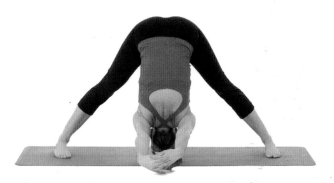

Full posture
• Follow steps 1–4, but keep your legs straight and your hands on the floor.

Moving on
• **Inhale** Come up to standing.
• **Exhale** Rest your hands on your waist ready to start the next posture.

Wide-legged Forward Bend D

Prasarita Padottanasana This is the last of the Prasarita Padottanasana variations.

Benefits

The forward bend continues to work on the flexibility of the back of the body and the shoulders. It also encourages bandha practice.

Contraindications

See page 46.

1 Inhale Draw back your shoulders and elbows to open your chest, as before.

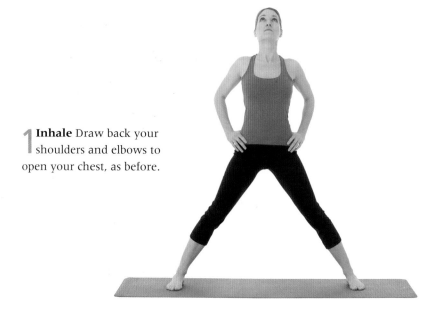

2 Exhale Bend your knees, fold forward and catch your big toes. If you are less flexible you may need to bring your feet slightly closer together to enable you to reach your toes.

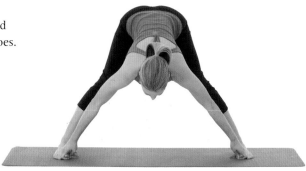

3 Inhale Maintaining the grip on your toes, look up.

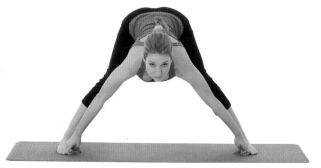

4 Exhale Take your head toward the floor. Look at your nose. Hold the posture for five breaths in and out.

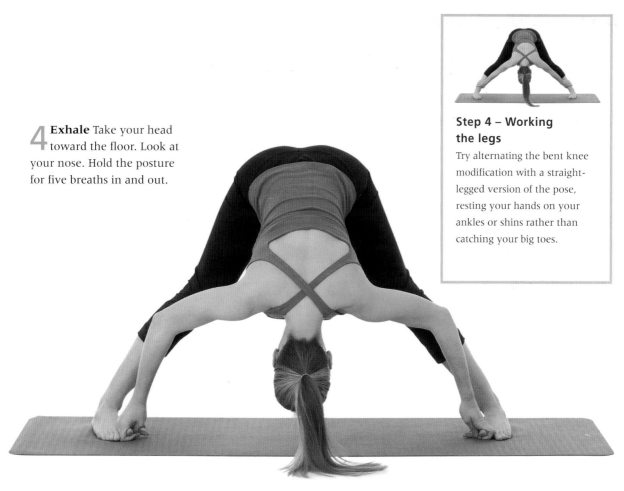

Step 4 – Working the legs

Try alternating the bent knee modification with a straight-legged version of the pose, resting your hands on your ankles or shins rather than catching your big toes.

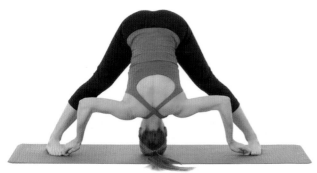

Full posture

• Follow steps 1–4, but make sure that your legs are straight and your head is on the floor.

Moving on

• **Inhale** Look up, maintaining the grip on your toes.
• **Exhale** Take your hands to your waist.
• **Inhale** Come up to standing.
• **Exhale** Step or jump back to Neutral Position, facing the front of the mat.

Lateral Forward Bend

Parsvottanasana After completing this posture, finish Lesson 3 with the breathing and relaxation in Lesson 15 (see pages 134–39).

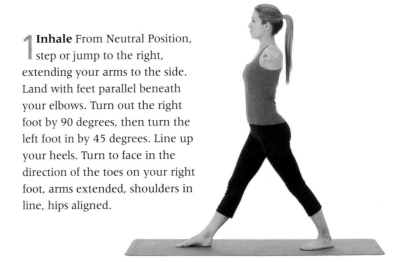

1 **Inhale** From Neutral Position, step or jump to the right, extending your arms to the side. Land with feet parallel beneath your elbows. Turn out the right foot by 90 degrees, then turn the left foot in by 45 degrees. Line up your heels. Turn to face in the direction of the toes on your right foot, arms extended, shoulders in line, hips aligned.

Benefits

Opens the shoulders and chest while lengthening and straightening the upper back.

Contraindications

See page 46.

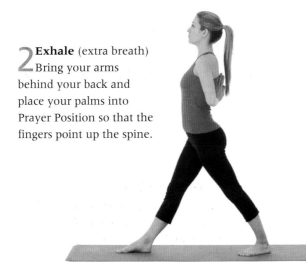

2 **Exhale** (extra breath) Bring your arms behind your back and place your palms into Prayer Position so that the fingers point up the spine.

Inhale (extra breath) Arch backward, opening the chest and shoulders. Take your hands higher, if possible, and press your palms and fingers together.

Step 2 – Alternative arm position

If you cannot bring your palms into Prayer Position, grasp opposite elbows with your hands instead.

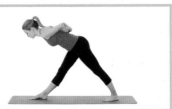

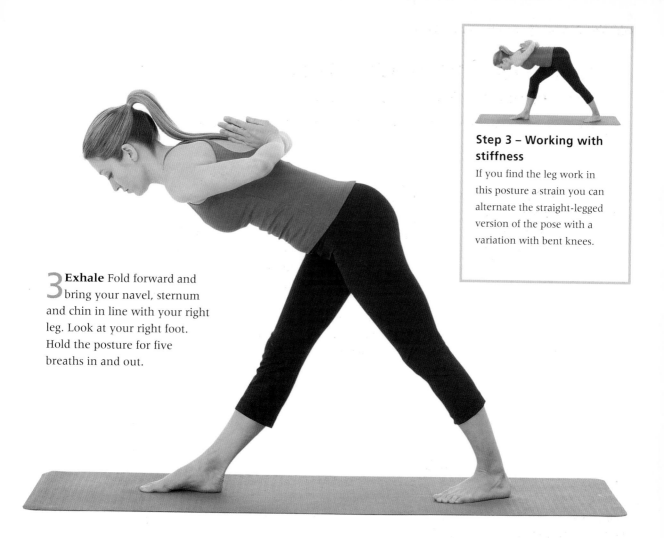

Step 3 – Working with stiffness

If you find the leg work in this posture a strain you can alternate the straight-legged version of the pose with a variation with bent knees.

3 **Exhale** Fold forward and bring your navel, sternum and chin in line with your right leg. Look at your right foot. Hold the posture for five breaths in and out.

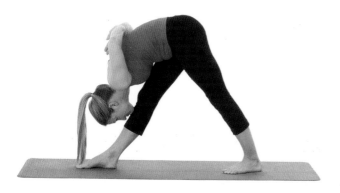

Full posture

• Work with both legs straight, your hips and shoulders squared forward. Take your navel, sternum and chin to touch your right leg.

Changing side

• **Inhale** Come up to standing. Change your feet so the left foot angles out by 90 degrees, your right foot by 45 degrees.
• **Exhale** Repeat the posture on the left.

Coming out

• **Inhale** Come up to standing. Bring the feet back to parallel.
• **Exhale** Step or jump back to Neutral Position, facing the front of the mat. Release your arms.

Lateral forward bend **67**

Modified Leg Balance

Utthita Hasta Padangusthasana Before starting this lesson, practise Lessons 1–3. Make sure you have memorized the previous sequences by heart before beginning this lesson.

> **Benefits**
>
> Both the modified and full posture (on pages 70–71) build strength, flexibility, balance and bandha control.
>
> **Contraindications**
>
> See page 46.

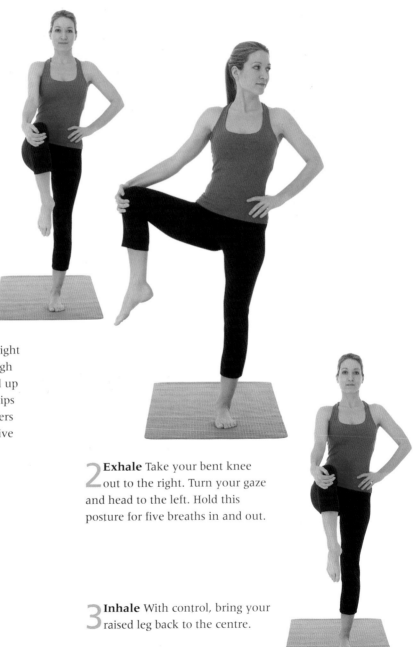

1 Inhale Stand in Neutral Position at the front of the mat. Balance on your left foot, taking your left hand to your waist. Bend your right knee and hold it with your right hand, keeping your right thigh parallel with the floor. Stand up straight, making sure your hips are aligned and your shoulders even. Hold this posture for five breaths in and out.

2 Exhale Take your bent knee out to the right. Turn your gaze and head to the left. Hold this posture for five breaths in and out.

3 Inhale With control, bring your raised leg back to the centre.

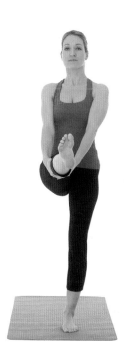

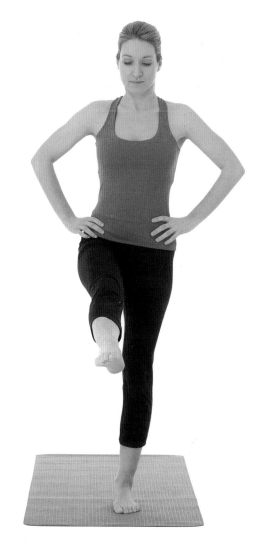

4 **Exhale** Hold beneath the thigh of your raised leg (if you are flexible, hold your ankle). Straighten your raised leg.

5 **Inhale** Take both hands to your waist, squeeze tight, and keep your foot raised as high as you can. Look at your foot. Hold this posture for five breaths in and out.

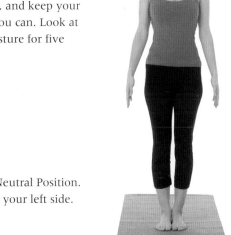

6 **Exhale** Return to Neutral Position. Repeat the steps on your left side.

Extended Leg Balance

Utthita Hasta Padangusthasana After practising the modified sequence for a few days, try the full posture, keeping your extended leg bent, if necessary. Eventually, you should be able to straighten both legs.

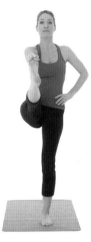

1 Inhale Stand in Neutral Position at the front of the mat. Balance on your left foot, taking your left hand to your waist. Lift your right leg, grasping the big toe with the first two fingers and thumbs of your right hand. Straighten your raised leg.

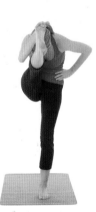

2 Exhale Fold forward over your extended leg, touching your chin to your right shin. Hold this posture for five breaths in and out.

3 Inhale Carefully come back upright, extending your spine to stand tall.

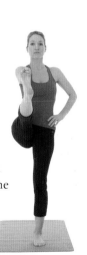

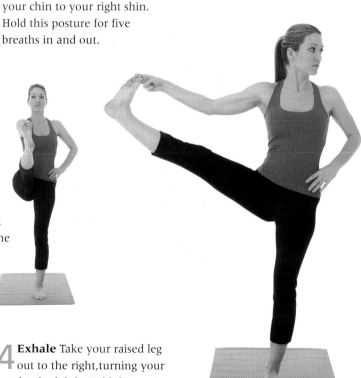

4 Exhale Take your raised leg out to the right, turning your head to look left. Hold this posture for five breaths in and out.

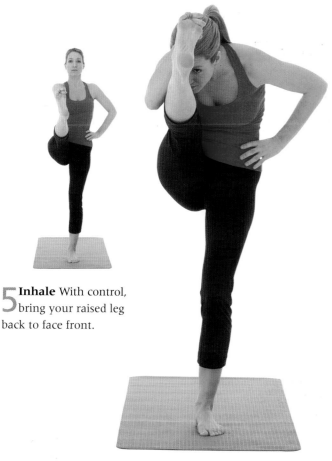

5 **Inhale** With control, bring your raised leg back to face front.

6 **Exhale** Fold forward over your raised leg, again touching your chin to your shin.

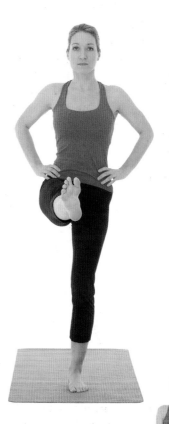

7 **Inhale** Come back upright, bringing your hands to your waist. Point your outstretched toes and keep your leg raised as high as possible. Hold this posture for five breaths in and out.

8 **Exhale** Lower your leg and come back to Neutral Position. Repeat the steps on your left side.

Standing Half-bound Lotus Forward Bend

Ardha Baddha Padmottanasana If you have a knee injury substitute Tree Posture (see contraindications). Finish your practice with Lesson 15 (see pages 134–39).

Benefits

Improves circulation to the spleen and liver. Opens the hips and improves balance.

Contraindications

Be careful if you have knee problems. Practise Tree Posture instead until any injury has healed: rest your raised foot on the inside of your opposite thigh and bring your hands into Prayer Position at your chest.

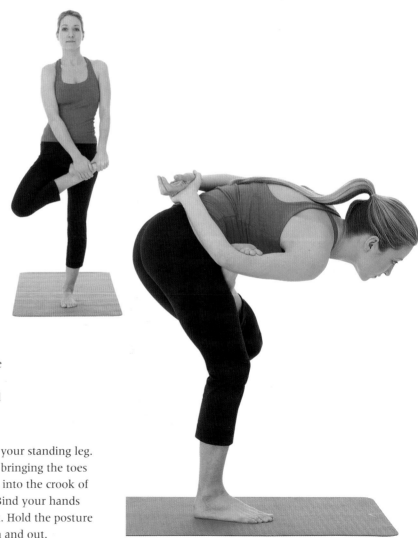

1 Inhale From Neutral Position, balance on your left foot. Take your right leg off the ground and bend the knee toward your chest. Holding your right knee with your right hand, your right foot with your left hand, gently guide your foot toward Lotus Position. The top of your right foot should rest on your left thigh.

2 Exhale Bend your standing leg. Fold forward, bringing the toes of your right foot into the crook of your left elbow. Bind your hands behind your back. Hold the posture for five breaths in and out.

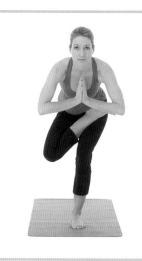

Step 2 – Working with stiffness

If you cannot bind your foot into the crook of your elbow, bring your hands into Prayer Position, bend your standing leg and lean forward to increase the stretch in the lotus hip.

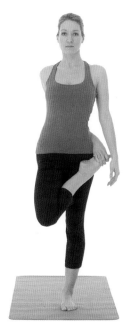

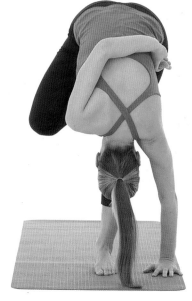

Full posture

• **Inhale** Bring the raised foot into Lotus Position.
• **Exhale** Twist to the right and bind the right foot with the right hand.

• **Inhale** Stand up straight, remaining bound.
• **Exhale** Extend forward, bringing your left hand to the floor and your chin toward your left shin. Look at your right foot.

Changing side

• **Inhale** Extend the spine. Look up.
• **Exhale** Bend the standing leg slightly.
• **Inhale** Come up to standing.
• **Exhale** Release to come back to Neutral Position. Repeat the steps on your left side.

Coming out

• **Inhale** Come back to Neutral Position, standing at the front of the mat.

Warrior Sequence

Utkatasana, Virabhadrasana A and B First practise Lessons 1 to 4, memorizing the sequences. This routine uses Sun Salutation movements to link the standing and sitting postures. You should, by now, have developed enough strength to attempt the full postures. Finish your practice with Lessons 11 (see pages 112–15) and 15 (see pages 134–39).

Benefits

Strengthens the spine, arms and legs and improves squatting. Holding the warrior postures strengthens the muscles of the arms and legs.

Contraindications

Take care not to lunge too deeply into the bent knee in Warrior postures. Pay attention to keeping the knee directly over the ankle.

1 Inhale Begin at Neutral Position at the front of your mat. Reach up with straight arms, bringing your palms together. Look up at your thumbs.

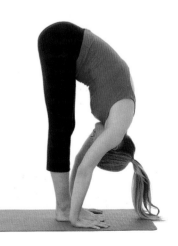

2 Exhale Fold forward from the hips and take your hands to the floor, shoulder distance apart. If you are stiff, keep your knees slightly bent in the forward bends. Tuck in your head and look at your nose.

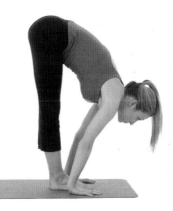

3 **Inhale** Arch back and open your chest, keeping your hands on the floor. Look up.

4 **Exhale** Step or jump your feet back, hip distance apart, into a push-up position. Bend your elbows to lower your chin 5 cm (2 in) from the floor, keeping your chest, pelvis and knees lifted from the floor. Look at your nose.

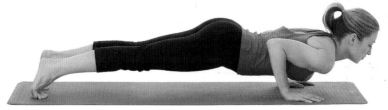

5 **Inhale** Straighten your arms, push your chest forward and roll over your toes into Upward Dog. Look at your nose.

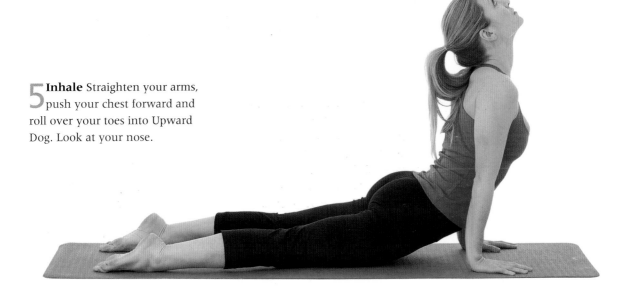

6 **Exhale** Push up your bottom and roll over your toes to come into Downward Dog. Look toward your navel.

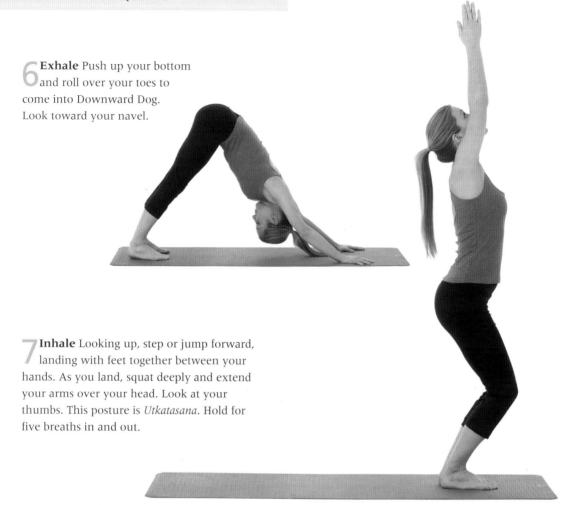

7 **Inhale** Looking up, step or jump forward, landing with feet together between your hands. As you land, squat deeply and extend your arms over your head. Look at your thumbs. This posture is *Utkatasana*. Hold for five breaths in and out.

Step 7 – Perfecting the pose

In *Utkatasana* (Seat of Power), you work in opposite directions, reaching down with your bottom and lifting up through your hands. Aim to bring your thighs parallel to the floor and your spine vertical. Straighten your back and arms and open your chest and shoulders.

8 **Exhale** Bring your hands to the floor while straightening the legs. Tuck your head in and look at your nose.

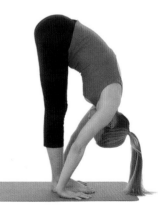

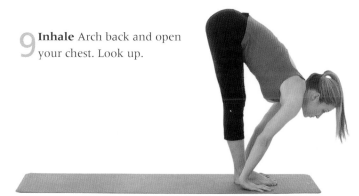

9 Inhale Arch back and open your chest. Look up.

10 Exhale Step or jump your feet back, hip distance apart, into a push-up position. Bend your elbows to lower your chin 5 cm (2 in) from the floor. Keep your chest, pelvis and knees lifted from the floor. Look at your nose.

11 Inhale Straighten your arms, push your chest forward and roll over your toes into Upward Dog. Look at your nose.

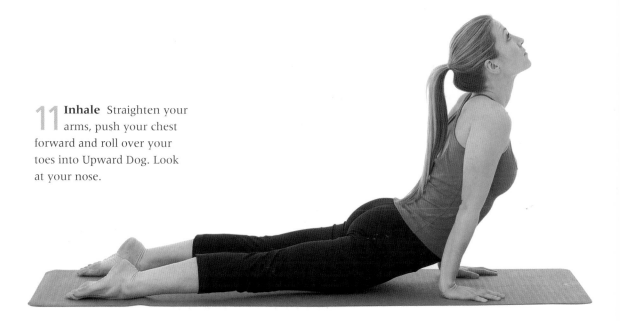

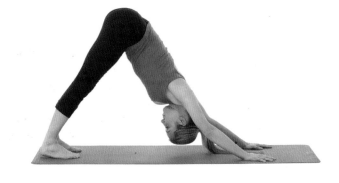

12 **Exhale** Push up your bottom and roll over your toes to come into Downward Dog. **Still exhaling** Turn the heel of your left foot in by 45 degrees and step your right foot between your hands. Keep your heels on the floor and aligned. Bend your right leg by 90 degrees so the knee is above the ankle. Keep your back leg straight.

13 **Inhale** Reach up and bring your palms together. Make sure your arms and spine are vertical, your hips and shoulders face evenly forward. Look up at your thumbs. Hold the posture for five breaths in and out.

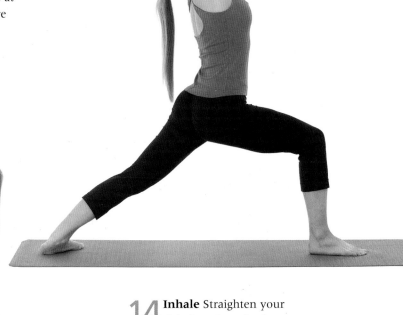

14 **Inhale** Straighten your right leg. Come back to centre, keeping the arms raised. Turn your right toes in and your left toes out. Turn your body 90 degrees to the left to face the other direction.

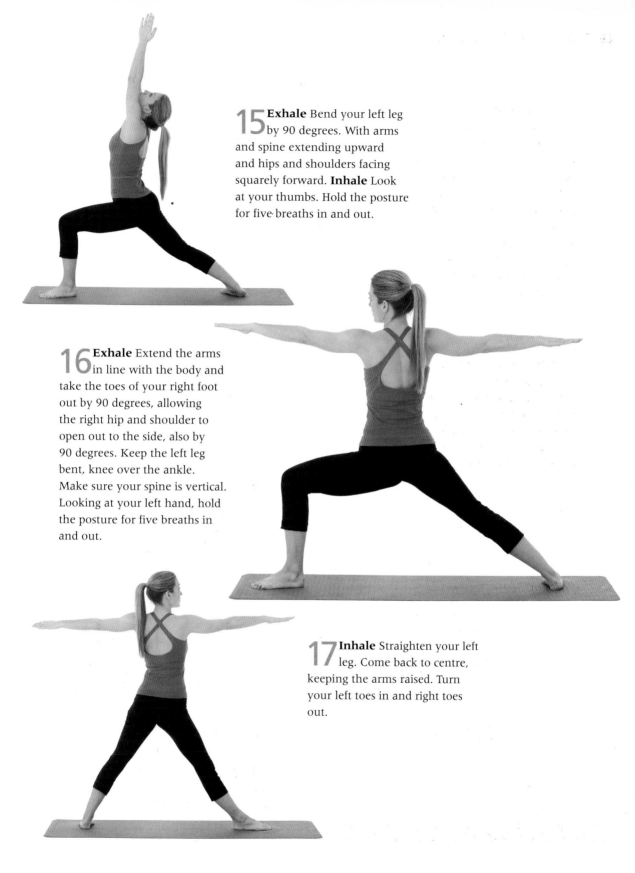

15 **Exhale** Bend your left leg by 90 degrees. With arms and spine extending upward and hips and shoulders facing squarely forward. **Inhale** Look at your thumbs. Hold the posture for five breaths in and out.

16 **Exhale** Extend the arms in line with the body and take the toes of your right foot out by 90 degrees, allowing the right hip and shoulder to open out to the side, also by 90 degrees. Keep the left leg bent, knee over the ankle. Make sure your spine is vertical. Looking at your left hand, hold the posture for five breaths in and out.

17 **Inhale** Straighten your left leg. Come back to centre, keeping the arms raised. Turn your left toes in and right toes out.

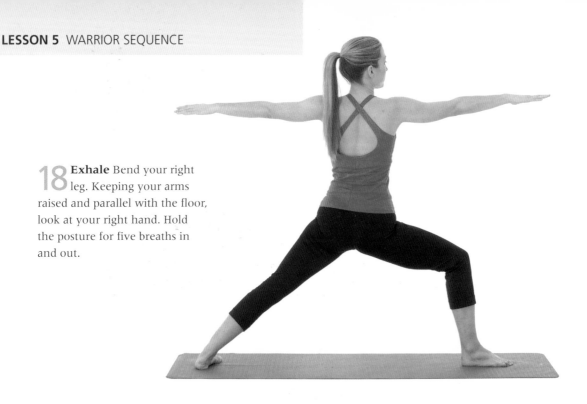

18 **Exhale** Bend your right leg. Keeping your arms raised and parallel with the floor, look at your right hand. Hold the posture for five breaths in and out.

19 **Inhale** Bring your hands to the floor, placed on either side of your right foot.

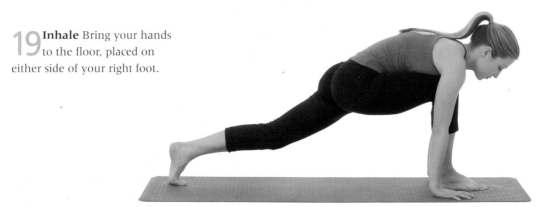

20 **Exhale** Step your feet back, hip distance apart, into a push-up position. Bend your elbows to lower your chin 5 cm (2 in) from the floor. Keep your chest, pelvis and knees raised from the floor. Look at your nose.

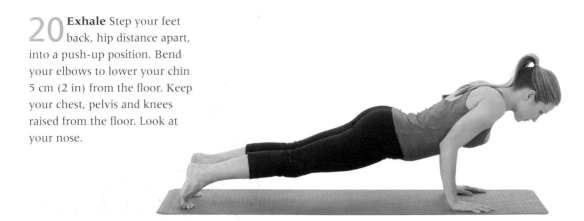

21 Inhale Straighten your arms, push your chest forward and roll over your toes into Upward Dog. Look at your nose.

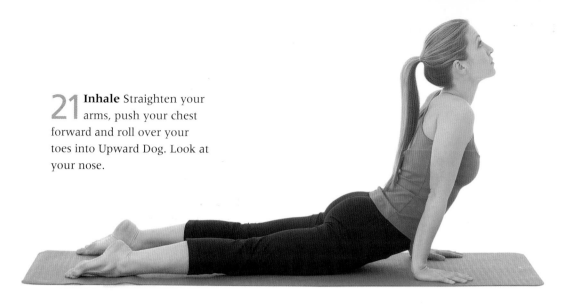

22 Exhale Push up your bottom and roll over your toes to come into Downward Dog.

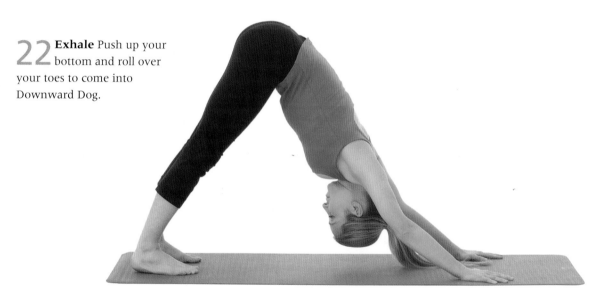

23 Inhale Jump your feet to, or through, your hands and sit down with legs extended straight in front of you.

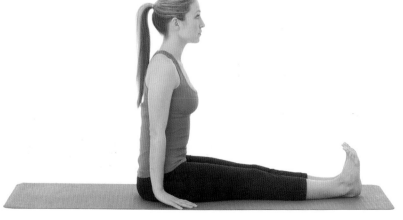

Sitting poses

Before starting this chapter, you should feel confident practising the previous lessons and be able to perform the postures and sequences in order without referring to the book. You are not expected to be able to do all the standing poses perfectly before attempting the sitting postures, but you should be confident with your breathing and bandhas, and be working toward the full posture. You should also be practising regularly (at least three times a week). There is nothing wrong with taking time to improve your standing postures. Be patient and persistent.

Lesson plan

Stage six
Lessons 1–5 (see pages 22–81)
Lesson 6 (see pages 84–91)
Lesson 11 (see pages 112–15)
Lesson 15 (see pages 134–39)

Stage seven
Lessons 1–6 (see pages 22–91)
Lesson 7 (see pages 92–95)
Lesson 11 (see pages 112–15)
Lesson 15 (see pages 134–39)

Stage eight
Lessons 1–7 (see pages 22–95)
Lesson 8 (see pages 96–101)
Lesson 11 (see pages 112–15)
Lesson 15 (see pages 134–39)

Stage nine
Lessons 1–8 (see pages 22–101)
Lesson 9 (see pages 102–107)
Lesson 11 (see pages 112–15)
Lesson 15 (see pages 134–39)

Stage ten
Lessons 1–9 (see pages 22–107)
Lesson 10 (see pages 108–109)
Lesson 11 (see pages 112–15)
Lesson 15 (see pages 134–39)

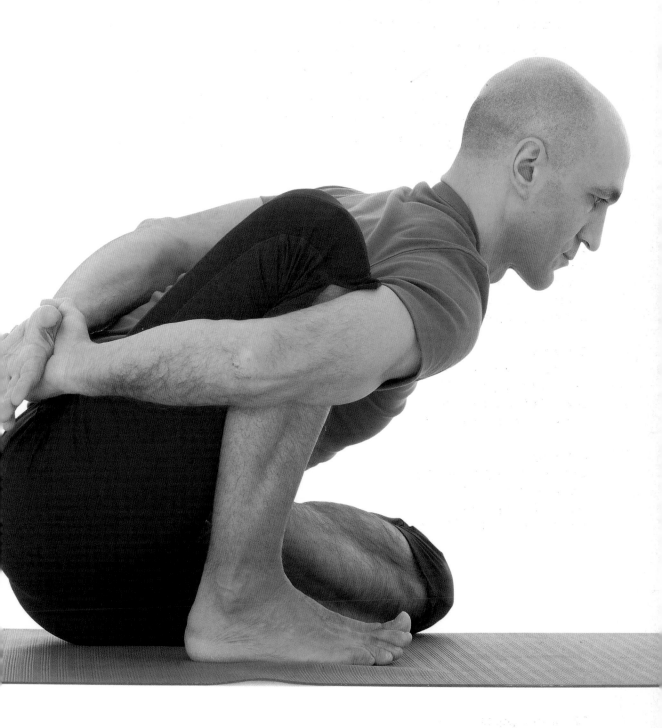

Seated Forward Bend

Paschimottanasana First, practise Lessons 1–5. This lesson introduces the basic sitting position, Staff Posture, before showing how to lengthen into *Paschimottanasana*, the first Seated Forward Bend.

Benefits

Prepares the body for correct forward bending by lengthening the spine and the back of the legs.

Contraindications

If you cannot reach your big toes, even when bending the knees slightly, spend longer in forward bends to allow the tendons in the muscles to release.

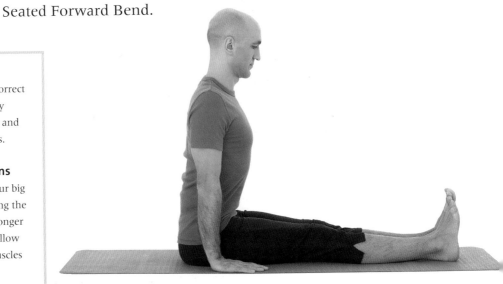

1 **Inhale** From the final Downward Dog in the Warrior Sequence, jump your feet to or through your hands and sit with your legs straight and your feet together. **Exhale** Sit up straight, lengthening your spine so that it is perpendicular to the floor. Press your palms to the floor on either side of your hips. Draw in your abdominal lock. Keep your feet vertical and pull up on your kneecaps and thighs to strengthen your knees. This is Staff Posture (*Dandasana*). Look at your toes while you hold the posture for five breaths in and out.

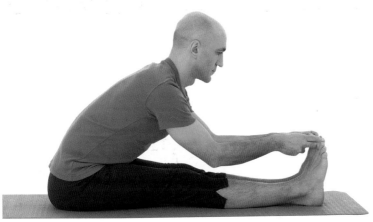

2 **Exhale** From Staff Posture, reach forward and grasp your big toes with the first two fingers and thumbs of each hand. If necessary bend your knees to catch your toes, keeping your knees and feet together.

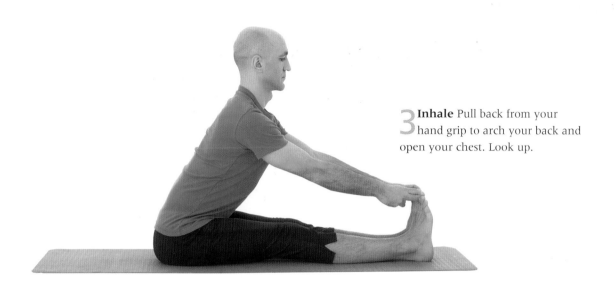

3 **Inhale** Pull back from your hand grip to arch your back and open your chest. Look up.

4 **Exhale** Fold forward, keeping the front and back of your body long. Look toward your feet. Hold the posture for five breaths in and out.

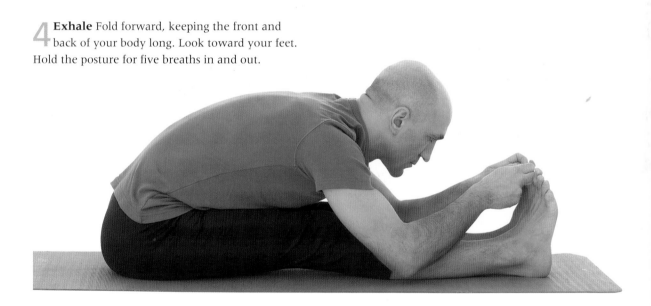

Step 4 – Working with stiffness

Focus on opening your chest, drawing back your shoulders and lengthening all the way from the lower back. If you have to bend your knees to reach your big toes, keep your feet and knees together so your legs stretch and develop evenly.

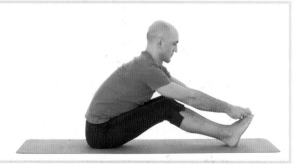

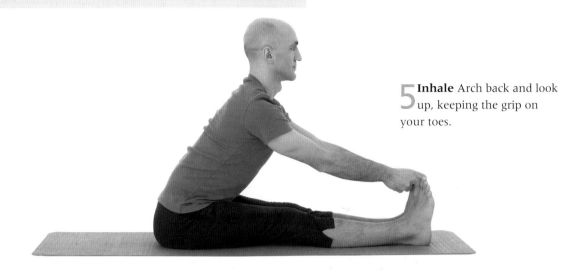

5 **Inhale** Arch back and look up, keeping the grip on your toes.

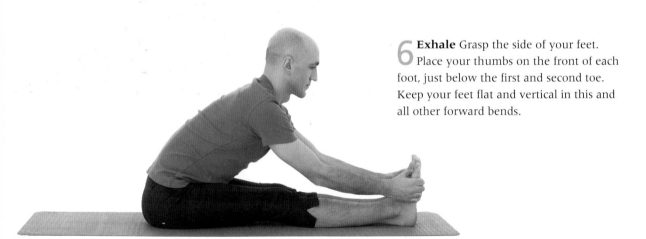

6 **Exhale** Grasp the side of your feet. Place your thumbs on the front of each foot, just below the first and second toe. Keep your feet flat and vertical in this and all other forward bends.

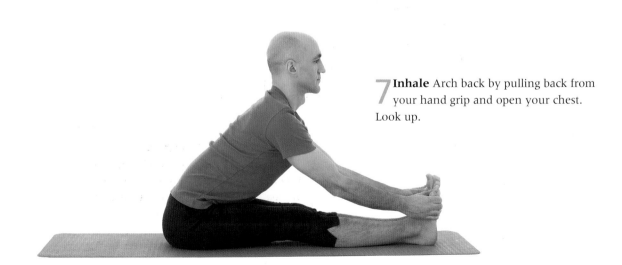

7 **Inhale** Arch back by pulling back from your hand grip and open your chest. Look up.

8 Exhale Fold forward, keeping the front and back of the body long. Looking toward your feet, hold the posture for five breaths.

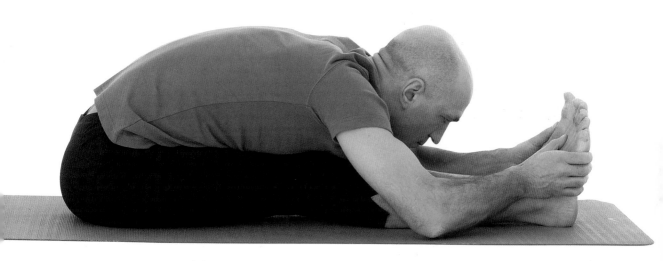

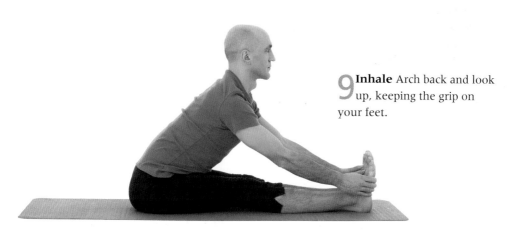

9 Inhale Arch back and look up, keeping the grip on your feet.

Coming out
• **Exhale** Release your hand grip and place your hands on the floor in front of your hips.

Step 9 – Perfecting the pose
In this and all subsequent forward bends, work first the belly to the thighs, then chest to knees, and finally chin between the shins. Do not drop your head – look toward your feet.

Linking Movement

Vinyasa The set of linking moves used between each posture is commonly known as a Vinyasa. When you see this word you are required to do the following movements.

Benefits
Keeps the body hot and flexible. Neutralizes the body between postures. Provides a back bend as a counterpose for the forward bends.

Contraindications
Do not jump if you have knee or back injuries. If you have a prolapsed disc or sciatica, take medical advice before practising.

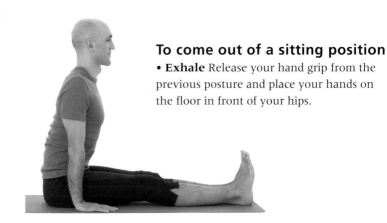

To come out of a sitting position
• **Exhale** Release your hand grip from the previous posture and place your hands on the floor in front of your hips.

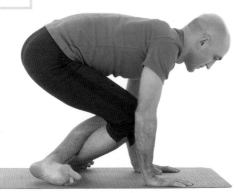

1 Inhale From sitting, cross your legs, roll forward, place your hands at the front of your mat and come onto hands and knees, ankles still crossed. Look up.

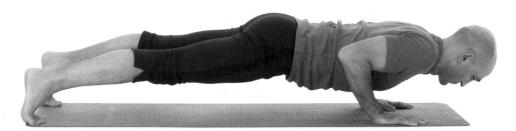

2 Exhale Step or jump your feet back, hip distance apart, into a push-up position. Bend your elbows to lower your chin 5 cm (2 in) from the floor. Keep your chest, pelvis and knees lifted from the mat. Look at your nose.

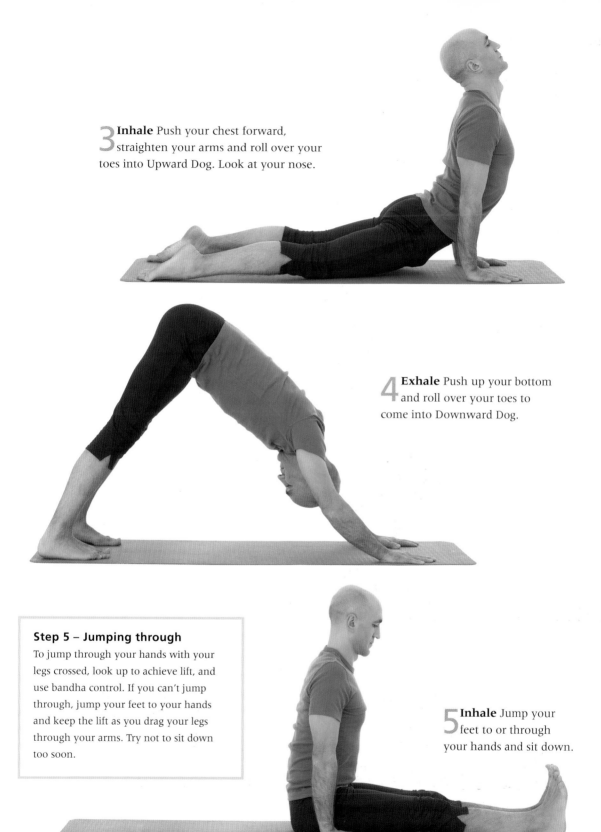

3 Inhale Push your chest forward, straighten your arms and roll over your toes into Upward Dog. Look at your nose.

4 Exhale Push up your bottom and roll over your toes to come into Downward Dog.

Step 5 – Jumping through

To jump through your hands with your legs crossed, look up to achieve lift, and use bandha control. If you can't jump through, jump your feet to your hands and keep the lift as you drag your legs through your arms. Try not to sit down too soon.

5 Inhale Jump your feet to or through your hands and sit down.

Seated Front Stretch

Purvattanasana If you're ready, move on to the next lesson
after completing this counterpose to the Seated Forward Bend.
Alternatively, finish your practice with Lessons 11 (see pages
112–15) and 15 (see pages 134–39).

Benefits	**Contraindications**
Strengthens the arms and wrists and the muscles along the back of the body. Encourages bandha control.	If you have neck injuries take extra care when moving the head back in this posture.

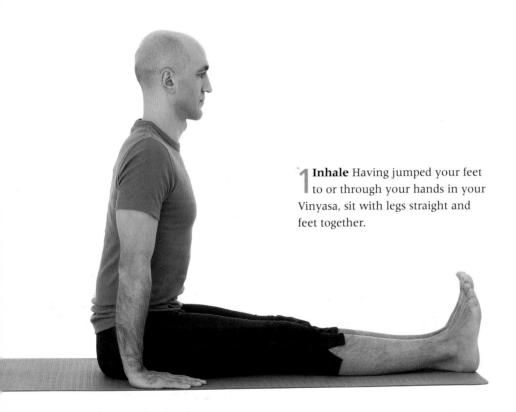

1 Inhale Having jumped your feet
to or through your hands in your
Vinyasa, sit with legs straight and
feet together.

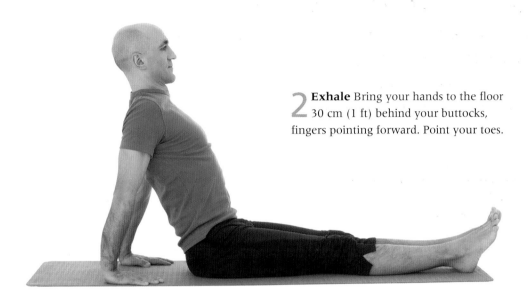

2 Exhale Bring your hands to the floor 30 cm (1 ft) behind your buttocks, fingers pointing forward. Point your toes.

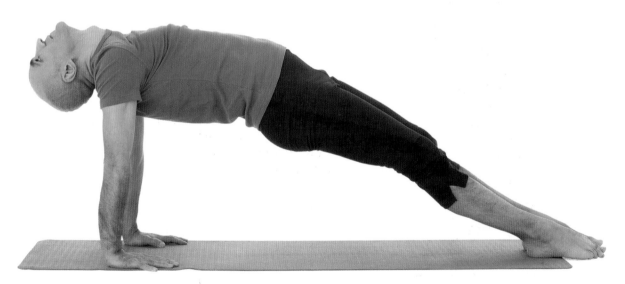

3 Inhale Lift your pelvis, abdomen and chest, keeping your legs straight. Lift your head back, maintaining length in the neck and look at your nose. Hold the posture for five breaths in and out.

Coming out
• **Exhale** Release down, bringing your hands to the floor in front of your hips.
• **Inhale** Do your Vinyasa.

Seated front stretch **91**

Seated Half-bound Lotus Forward Bend

Ardha Baddha Padma Paschimottanasana First, practise Lessons 1–6. Complete the Vinyasa from the last lesson to bring you into the starting position for this posture.

> **Benefits**
>
> Eases sciatica. Massages the liver and spleen.
>
> **Contraindications**
>
> Work with care and take advice from an experienced yoga teacher or medical professional if you experience pain in the knees.

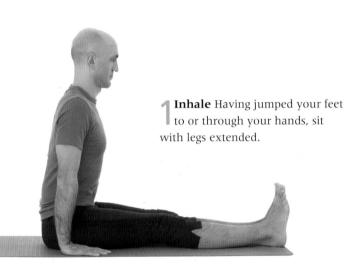

1 Inhale Having jumped your feet to or through your hands, sit with legs extended.

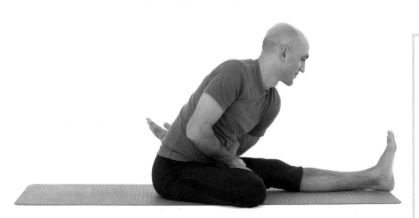

2 Exhale (you may need extra breaths) Bend your right knee. Aim to bring your right heel to press into the lower left abdomen. Place your right ankle on your left thigh, lined up with your left kneecap. This is Half-lotus Position. Fold forward, bringing the crook of your left elbow beneath your right foot. Reach behind your back with your left hand, palm facing upward.

> **Step 2 – Working with stiffness**
>
> In Lotus Position, the ankle must be supported by the opposite thigh rather than falling between your legs. If you feel pain in the foot or thigh, take your foot higher. Do not place the foot so far over that the ankle crosses the mid-line of the supporting leg. If in doubt, just practise the foot position gently and don't attempt the binding or forward bend.

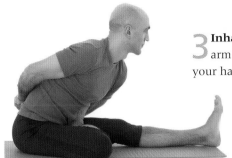

3 **Inhale** Sit upright and take your right arm behind your back. Bind (catch) your hands. Arch your back and look up.

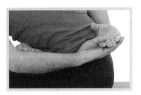

Back view

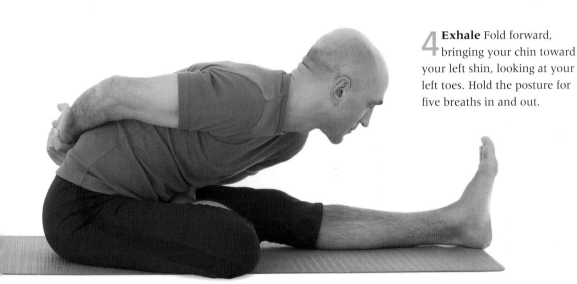

4 **Exhale** Fold forward, bringing your chin toward your left shin, looking at your left toes. Hold the posture for five breaths in and out.

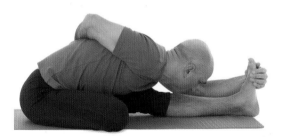

Changing side
• **Inhale** Keeping your grip on your hands behind you, arch backward and look up.
• **Exhale** Release your hands and Lotus leg, then extend your legs straight out in front. Repeat on the left side.

Coming out
• **Inhale** Arch backward and look up.
• **Exhale** Release the posture, bringing your hands to the floor in front of your hips.
• **Inhale** Do your Vinyasa.

Full posture
• **Inhale** Bring your right foot into Lotus Position.
• **Exhale** Bind your right foot with your right hand.
• **Inhale** Catch your left foot with your left hand, arch back and look up.
• **Exhale** Forward bend, looking at your extended foot.

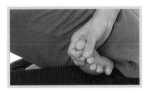

Back view

Seated half-bound lotus forward bend **93**

Transverse Bent-Knee Forward Bend

Tiriangmukhaikapada Paschimottanasana Come into the starting position from your last Vinyasa. After finishing the posture move on, if you are ready, to the next lesson or finish your practice with Lessons 11 (see pages 112–15) and 15 (see pages 134–39).

Benefits

The intense stretch in the buttocks and lower back can be helpful with sciatica. Opens the hips.

Contraindications

Be careful and take advice from an experienced yoga teacher or medical professional if you experience pain in the knees.

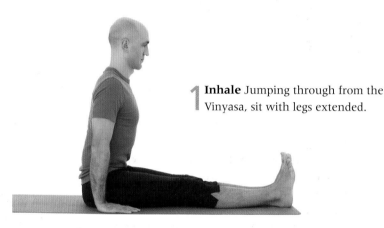

1 Inhale Jumping through from the Vinyasa, sit with legs extended.

2 Exhale Pull your calf muscle out of the way and bend your right knee. Bring your right foot alongside your right hip, toes pointing backward and sole of the foot facing the ceiling. Keep your knees close together.

3 Inhale Keeping your left hand on the floor for balance, reach forward to grasp the inside of your extended foot with your right hand. Arch the back and look up.

Step 3 – Perfecting the pose

In this posture, as in all forward bends, remember to keep your extended foot straight and vertical.

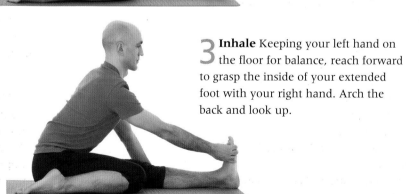

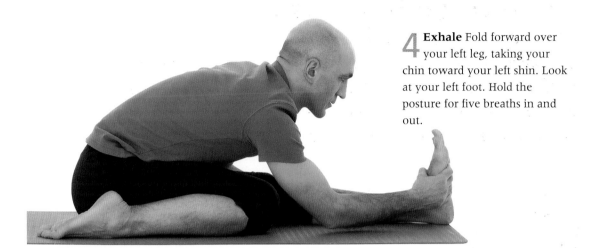

4 Exhale Fold forward over your left leg, taking your chin toward your left shin. Look at your left foot. Hold the posture for five breaths in and out.

Step 4 – Finding balance

It is normal to be out of balance to begin with. Remember to pull the calf muscle out of the way and adjust your buttocks so both sitting bones are flat on the floor. Some people find it helpful to place a pillow or book beneath the buttock of the extended leg. Try this if necessary, but bear in mind that props are not generally recommended in Ashtanga Yoga. You may also ease into posture using both hands as stabilizers.

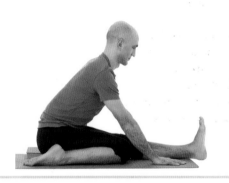

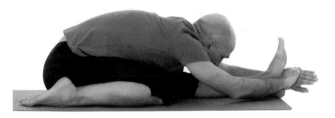

Full posture

• **Inhale** Jump through from the Vinyasa with your right knee bent into position and sit.
• **Exhale** Fold forward and bind your extended foot.
• **Inhale** Arch backward and look up.
• **Exhale** Forward bend, looking toward your front foot.

Changing side

• **Inhale** Arch backward and look up.
• **Exhale** Release the posture, bringing your hands to the floor in front of your hips. Repeat on the left side

Coming out

• **Inhale** Arch backward and look up.
• **Exhale** Release the posture, bringing your hands to the floor in front of your hips
• **Inhale** Do your Vinyasa.

Bent-Knee Forward Bend A

Janu Sirsasana A Before starting this lesson, complete Lessons 1–7 and do your Vinyasa.

Benefits
Opens the hips.

Contraindications
Work with care and take advice from an experienced yoga teacher or medical professional if you experience pain in the knees.

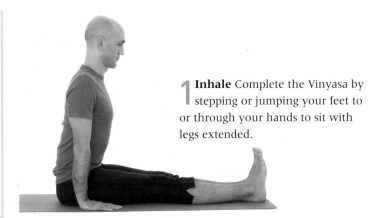

1 Inhale Complete the Vinyasa by stepping or jumping your feet to or through your hands to sit with legs extended.

Step 2 – Working with stiffness
Bring the foot as close to the groin as possible, and make sure the sole of the foot faces upward. If you feel pain in the bent knee, try elevating your knee by placing padding underneath, or by taking your foot further away from the groin.

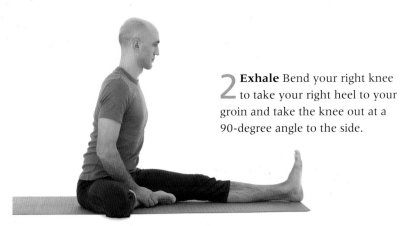

2 Exhale Bend your right knee to take your right heel to your groin and take the knee out at a 90-degree angle to the side.

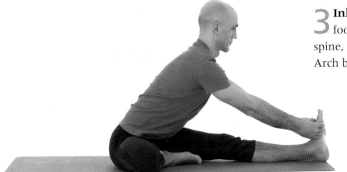

3 Inhale Reach for your left ankle or foot with both hands and extend your spine, aligning your shoulders and hips. Arch backward and look up.

4 **Exhale** Fold forward from the hips, straightening your extended leg. Look at your left foot. Hold the posture for five breaths in and out.

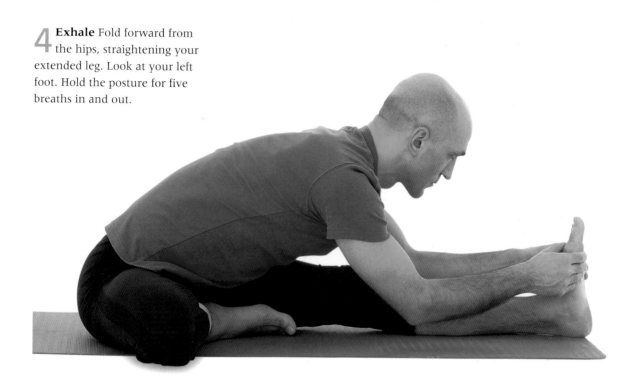

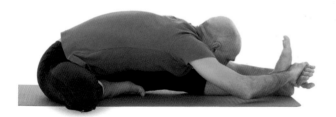

Full posture

• **Inhale** Jump through to sitting.
• **Exhale** Bend your right knee and bring your heel into the groin, as above.
• **Inhale** Grasp the wrist of your left hand around your left foot. Arch backward and look up.
• **Exhale** Fold forward, looking toward your front foot.

Changing side

• **Inhale** Arch backward and look up.
• **Exhale** Release your hands and repeat the posture on the left side.

Coming out

• **Inhale** Arch backward and look up.
• **Exhale** Release the posture, bringing your hands to the floor in front of your hips.
• **Inhale** Do your Vinyasa and move on to the next posture.

Bent-Knee Forward Bend B

Janu Sirsasana B At first this pose may hurt the ankle you are
sitting on. Use a towel for padding until you toughen up.

Benefits

Stretches and strengthens the
ankles. Encourages the
practice of Mula Bandha,
helpful to tone the pelvic
floor. In men, helps prevent
problems with the
prostate gland.

Contraindications

See page 96. If the position
causes pressure in the knees,
work gently.

1 Inhale (extra breath) Complete the
Vinyasa by stepping or jumping your
feet to or through your hands to sit with
legs extended.

2 Exhale (extra breath) Bend your right
leg to bring your right heel to your
groin and the knee out 85 degrees to the
side.

3 Inhale Place your hands on the
floor on either side of your hips
and lift yourself up and forward until
your right heel is beneath your anus.

4 Exhale Sit your anus onto the heel so your
buttocks are raised from the ground. If you
are stiff, your toes may need to point out to the
side rather than forward as pictured.

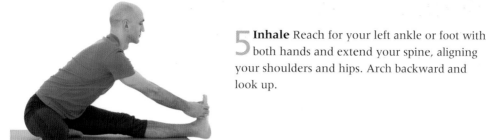

5 **Inhale** Reach for your left ankle or foot with both hands and extend your spine, aligning your shoulders and hips. Arch backward and look up.

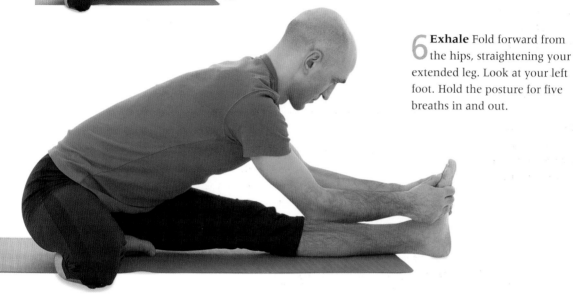

6 **Exhale** Fold forward from the hips, straightening your extended leg. Look at your left foot. Hold the posture for five breaths in and out.

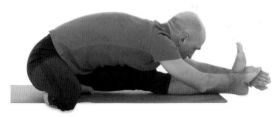

Full posture
• **Inhale** Jump through to sitting.
• **Exhale** Bend the right knee and bring your heel beneath your anus. Sit down.
• **Inhale** Grasp the wrist of your left hand around your left foot. Arch backward and look up.
• **Exhale** Fold forward, looking toward your front foot.

Changing side
• **Inhale** Arch backward and look up.
• **Exhale** Release your hands and repeat the posture on the left side.

Coming out
• **Inhale** Arch backward and look up.
• **Exhale** Release the posture, bringing your hands to the floor in front of your hips.
• **Inhale** Do your Vinyasa and move on to the next posture.

Bent-Knee Forward Bend C

Janu Sirsasana C After completing this pose, move onto the
next lesson if you feel ready, or finish your practice with Lessons
11 (see pages 112–15) and 15 (see pages 134–39).

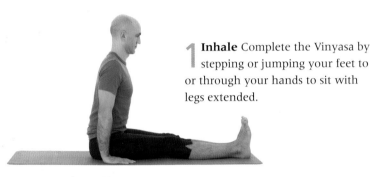

Benefits
Massages the uterus. May
encourage the breakdown of
fibroids. Stimulates the
pancreas.

Contraindications
See page 96 and work
cautiously if you have pain in
your knees.

1 **Inhale** Complete the Vinyasa by
stepping or jumping your feet to
or through your hands to sit with
legs extended.

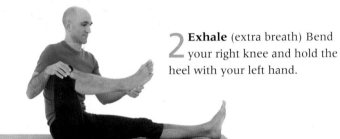

2 **Exhale** (extra breath) Bend
your right knee and hold the
heel with your left hand.

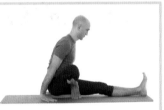

Step 4 – Stretching further
To find extra stretch in your
toes, bring your hands to the
floor on either side of your
hips and lift yourself up and
slightly forward so your
weight is in the ball of the
right foot. Gently ease the
knee toward the floor. You can
use a book to sit on if you find
this difficult. If you wish,
remain in this position until
you are ready to go further.

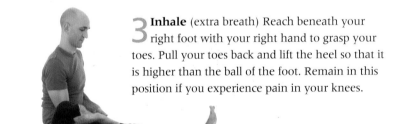

3 **Inhale** (extra breath) Reach beneath your
right foot with your right hand to grasp your
toes. Pull your toes back and lift the heel so that it
is higher than the ball of the foot. Remain in this
position if you experience pain in your knees.

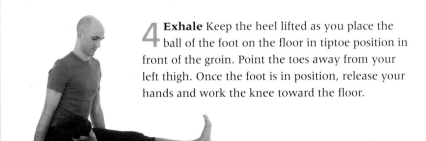

4 **Exhale** Keep the heel lifted as you place the
ball of the foot on the floor in tiptoe position in
front of the groin. Point the toes away from your
left thigh. Once the foot is in position, release your
hands and work the knee toward the floor.

5 **Inhale** Reach for your left ankle or foot with both hands and extend the spine, aligning shoulders and hips. Arch backward and look up.

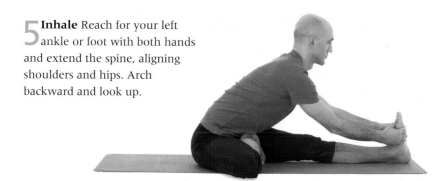

6 **Exhale** Fold forward from the hips, straightening your extended leg. Look at your left foot. Hold the posture for five breaths in and out.

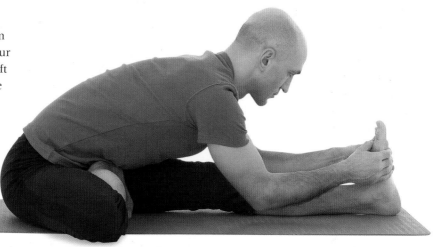

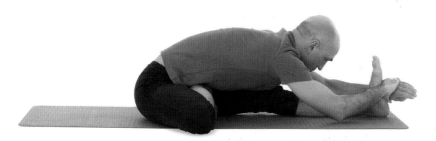

Full posture
• **Inhale** Jump through to sitting.
• **Exhale** Bend the right knee and bring the foot into position.
• **Inhale** Grasp the wrist of your left hand around your left foot. Arch backward and look up.
• **Exhale** Fold forward, looking toward your left foot.

Changing side
• **Inhale** Arch backward and look up.
• **Exhale** Release and repeat the posture on the left side.

Coming out
• **Inhale** Arch backward and look up.
• **Exhale** Release the posture, then bring your hands to the floor in front of your hips.
• **Inhale** Do your Vinyasa.

Posture of the Sage A

Marichyasana A Before starting this lesson, complete Lessons 1–8 and do your Vinyasa.

> ### Benefits
> Opens the hips and prepares for leg-behind-the-head postures.
>
> ### Contraindications
> None.

1 **Inhale** Complete your Vinyasa by stepping or jumping your feet to or through your hands and sit with legs extending forward. Bend your right knee and bring your right foot flat to the floor, ankle in line with the outside of the left hip.

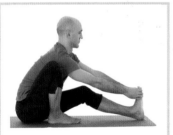

Step 2 – Learning to bind

Make sure you leave enough space between your left thigh and right foot to bring your torso forward. Keep the outer edge of your bent-leg foot parallel to your extended leg. If you are unable to bind your hands behind your back, reach forward with both hands and hold the extended foot before bending forward.

2 **Exhale** Fold forward with your right arm extended and wrap your arm around your right shin, reaching back to bind (catch) your left hand behind your back.

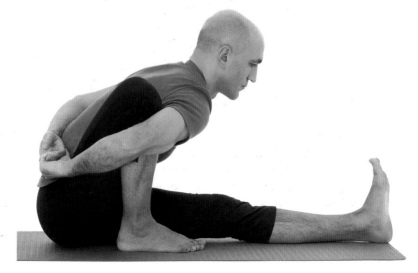

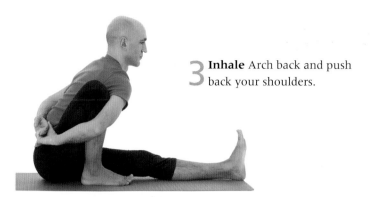

3 **Inhale** Arch back and push back your shoulders.

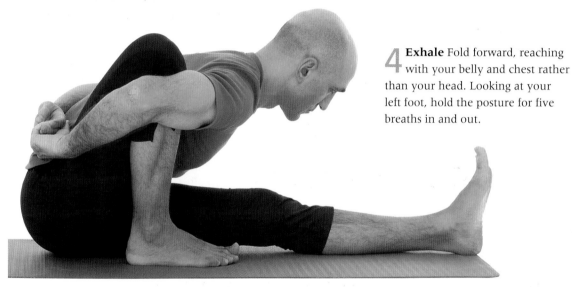

4 **Exhale** Fold forward, reaching with your belly and chest rather than your head. Looking at your left foot, hold the posture for five breaths in and out.

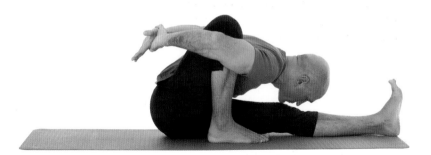

Full posture
• **Exhale** Fold forward, this time taking your chin to the extended shin. Clasp your opposite wrist with the hand that wraps around the knee. Keep your arms long and torso extended.

Changing side
• **Inhale** Arch backward.
• **Exhale** Release, and repeat the posture on the left side.

Coming out
• **Inhale** Arch backward and look up.
• **Exhale** Release the posture, and bring your hands to the floor in front of your hips.
• **Inhale** Do your Vinyasa.

Posture of the Sage B

Marichyasana B When you feel ready, move onto the next
lesson, or finish your practice with Lessons 11 (see pages 112–15)
and 15 (see pages 134–39).

Benefits

Massages the digestive system
and female reproductive
organs.

Contraindications

In Lotus Position variations
never push into knee pain. If
necessary, take the advice of a
physiotherapist or knee
specialist.

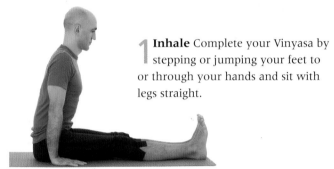

1 Inhale Complete your Vinyasa by
stepping or jumping your feet to
or through your hands and sit with
legs straight.

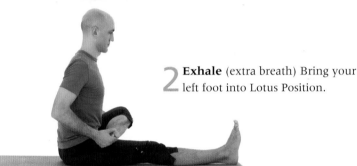

2 Exhale (extra breath) Bring your
left foot into Lotus Position.

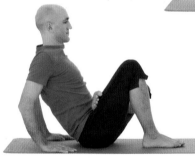

3 Inhale (extra breath) Place
your hands on the floor behind
your back and lean backward. Bend
your right leg vertically and bring
the foot flat on the floor to line up
the ankle and the outside of the
right hip.

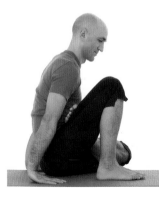

4 Exhale (extra breath) Sit upright and
lean to the left, lifting your right buttock
off the floor and bringing your left knee
to the mat. Keep the right knee vertical.
If necessary, remain in this position for
five or more breaths. Don't attempt
any arm movements until this sitting
position is comfortable.

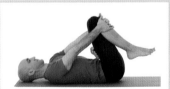

Step 4 – Working with stiffness

You are not alone if you find
this leg position challenging.
Practise opening the hips by
lying back with the left foot in
Lotus Position. Hug your right
knee toward your chest until
you are ready to attempt the
sitting position.

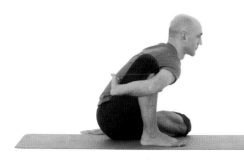

5 **Inhale** (extra breath) Keep your left hand on the floor for balance. Reach backward with your right arm and wedge the elbow in front of your right shin. Arch backward and look up.

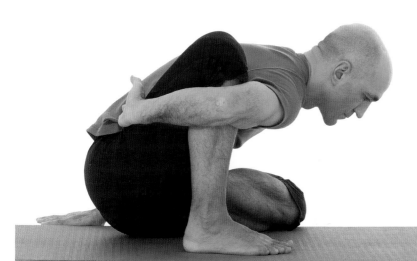

6 **Exhale** Work toward a forward bend, attempting to bring your head to the floor between your foot and your knee. Looking at your nose, hold the posture for five breaths in and out. You may try binding your hands if you feel more comfortable in this posture.

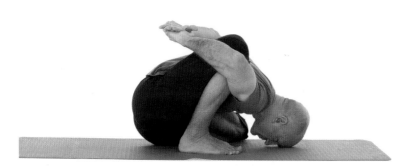

Full posture
• **Inhale** Set the leg position and wrap your arms around your vertical knee with wrist bound behind the back, as in Posture of the Sage A.
• **Exhale** Fold forward.

Changing side
• **Inhale** Arch backward.
• **Exhale** Release arms and legs, and repeat the posture on the left side.

Coming out
• **Inhale** Arch backward and look up.
• **Exhale** Release the posture, and bring your hands to the floor in front of your hips.
• **Inhale** Do your Vinyasa.

Posture of the Sage C

Marichyasana C Don't start this lesson until you feel
comfortable with Lessons 1–8; do your Vinyasa before beginning.

Benefits

Twists relieve backache, headache, stiff necks and shoulders. They improve spinal flexibility and open the hips while stimulating digestion by massaging internal organs. Breathing under pressure helps expand the lungs.

Contraindications

Don't practise twists after stomach operations. Take medical advice if you have a hernia.

1 **Inhale** Complete your Vinyasa by stepping or jumping your feet to or through your hands and sit with legs straight. Bend your right leg and bring your right foot flat to the floor. Line up the outer edge of the foot with the outside of your left hip. Sit up straight.

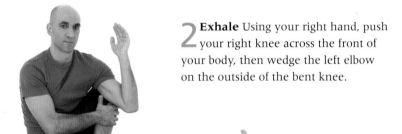

2 **Exhale** Using your right hand, push your right knee across the front of your body, then wedge the left elbow on the outside of the bent knee.

3 **Inhale** Keeping your left elbow wedged on the outside of your right knee, place your right hand on the floor behind your bottom. Extend the spine.

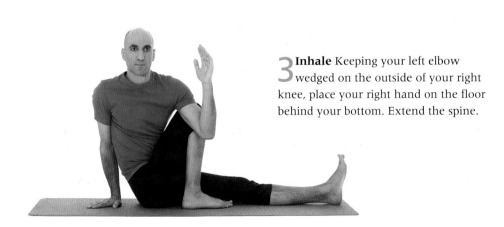

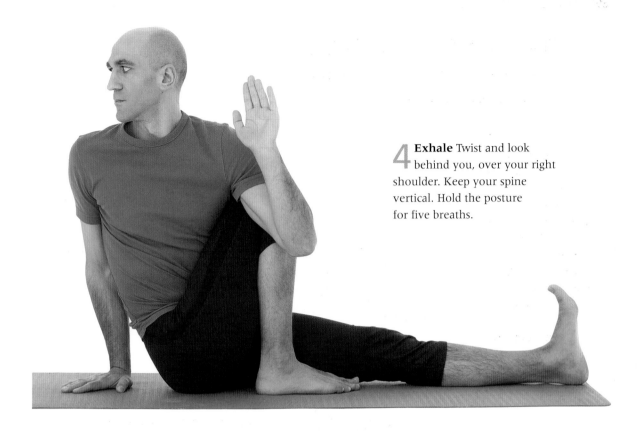

4 **Exhale** Twist and look behind you, over your right shoulder. Keep your spine vertical. Hold the posture for five breaths.

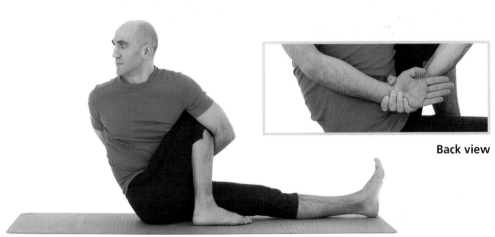

Back view

Full posture
• Wedge your left elbow on the outside of your right knee, then wrap your arm around the leg and bind your right hand or wrist behind your back. Extend the spine and open your shoulders.

Changing side
• **Inhale** Look forward.
• **Exhale** Release your arms and legs, and repeat the posture on the left side.

Coming out
• **Inhale** Look forward.
• **Exhale** Release the posture, and bring your hands to the floor.
• **Inhale** Do your Vinyasa.

Boat Posture

Navasana Finish the session with Lessons 11 (see pages 112–15)
and 15 (see pages 134–39). Once you are able to hold five sets of
Boat Posture, proceed to Chapter Three, Finishing Poses.

Benefits

Strengthens the hips, back
and abdominal muscles.
Encourages bandha control.

Contraindications

Take medical advice before
practising if you have a hernia
or back problems.

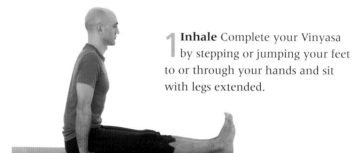

1 **Inhale** Complete your Vinyasa
by stepping or jumping your feet
to or through your hands and sit
with legs extended.

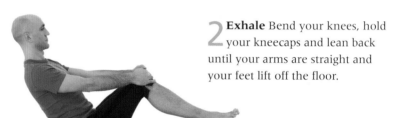

2 **Exhale** Bend your knees, hold
your kneecaps and lean back
until your arms are straight and
your feet lift off the floor.

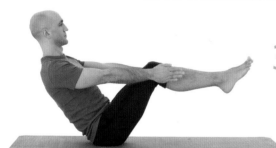

3 **Inhale** Release your hands, bring the
palms to face your knees.

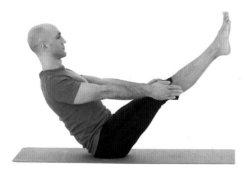

4 **Exhale** Straighten your
legs. Bring your legs and
spine each to 45 degrees
from the floor, arms parallel
to the floor and each other.
Keep your shoulders and
back straight. Hold the
posture for five breaths.

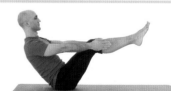

Step 4 – Perfecting the pose

In this pose, you must hold the spine
and thighs at the correct angle. If
you cannot straighten your legs
without your back and chest
collapsing, practise with knees bent.

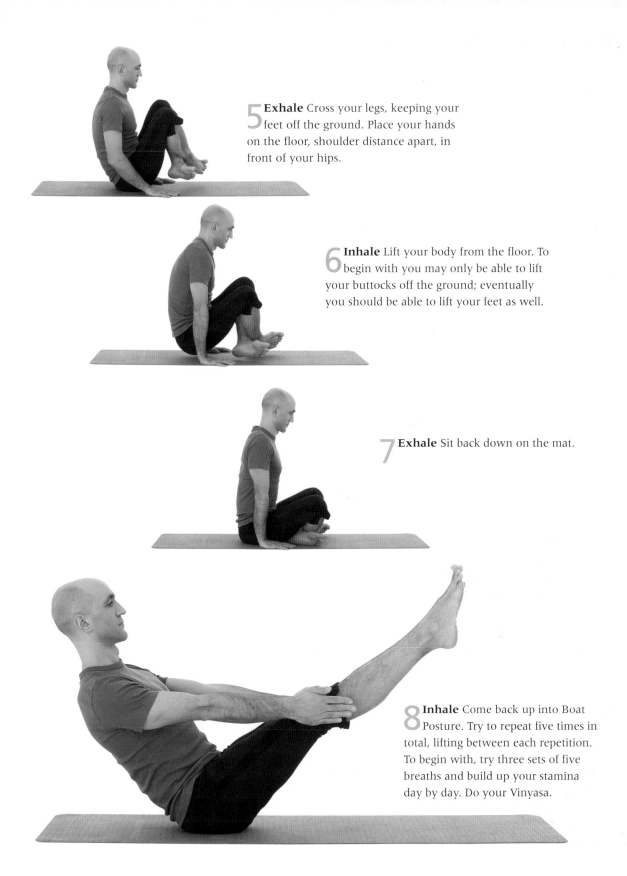

5 Exhale Cross your legs, keeping your feet off the ground. Place your hands on the floor, shoulder distance apart, in front of your hips.

6 Inhale Lift your body from the floor. To begin with you may only be able to lift your buttocks off the ground; eventually you should be able to lift your feet as well.

7 Exhale Sit back down on the mat.

8 Inhale Come back up into Boat Posture. Try to repeat five times in total, lifting between each repetition. To begin with, try three sets of five breaths and build up your stamina day by day. Do your Vinyasa.

Boat posture **109**

Finishing poses

When you first start learning Ashtanga Yoga, you finish your practice with the breathing sequence in Lesson 15, then relax for 10–30 minutes. As you become more advanced in your practice, so too do the finishing postures. After completing the standing postures in Lessons 1–5 you will be ready to learn the back bends in Lesson 11. Once you have learned the sitting postures up to Boat Posture in Lessons 6–10, you can add Shoulder Stand and Head Stand to your finishing sequence. Do not practise these postures out of sequence, nor attempt them before you're ready. Shoulder Stand and Head Stand in particular require a certain degree of flexibility for safe practice.

Lesson plan

Stage 11
Lessons 1–10 (see pages 22–109)
Lesson 11 (see pages 112–15)
Lesson 12 (see pages 116–19)
Lesson 15 (see pages 134–39)

Stage 12
Lessons 1–10 (see pages 22–109)
Lesson 11 (see pages 112–15)
Lesson 13 (see pages 120–27)
Lesson 15 (see pages 134–39)

Stage 13
Lessons 1–10 (see pages 22–109)
Lesson 11 (see pages 112–15)
Lesson 13 (see pages 120–27)
Lesson 14 (see pages 128–33)
Lesson 15 (see pages 134–39)

Stage 14
Lessons 1–10 (see pages 22–109)
Lesson 11 (see pages 112–15)
Lesson 13 (see pages 120–27)
Lesson 14 (see pages 128–33)
Lesson 15 (see pages 134–39)

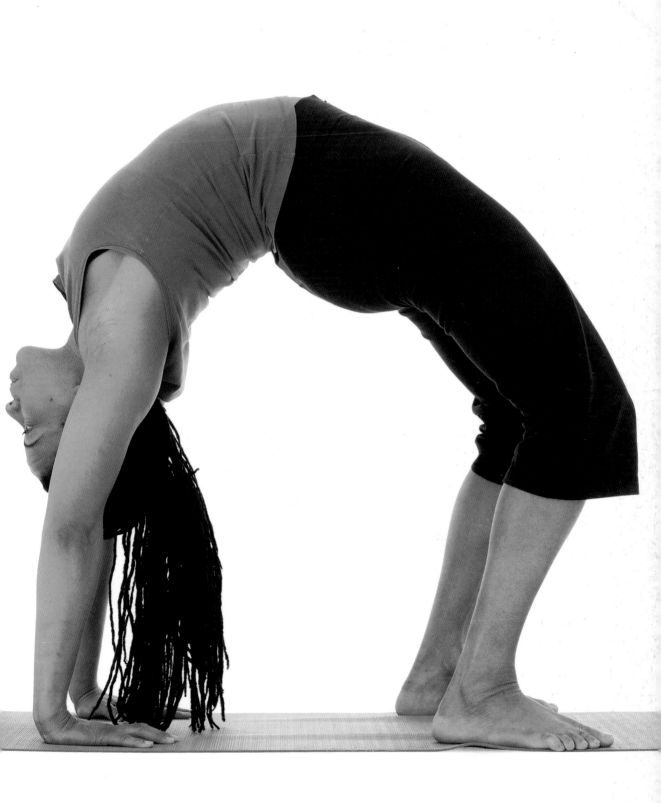

Face-up Bow

Urdhva Dhanurasana Before practising the postures in this
lesson you must have completed Lesson 5 (see pages 74–81): do
your practice to the end of the Warrior Sequence, then begin the
work here. Note that in back bends you inhale to lift into the
bend, exhaling to come down. Follow the Face-up Bow with the
Seated Forward Bend counterpose (see page 115). Then, if you are
ready, move on to the next lesson. Alternatively, come into the
appropriate sitting posture for the breathing sequence in Lesson 15
(see pages 134–39).

Benefits	Contraindications
Strengthens the arms and shoulders, makes the spine and shoulders more flexible. Anti-depressant properties.	May not be suitable for those with heart problems, high blood pressure, a bad back or injured knees. May also be beneficial for all of the above, depending on the degree of severity. If in doubt, seek medical advice or speak to a yoga therapist.

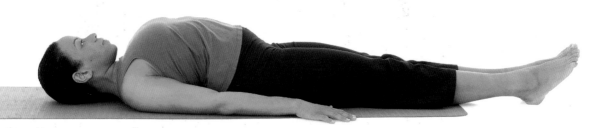

1 Inhale From the linking movement,
step or jump through to sitting as
usual, then lie down. Tuck your thumbs
beneath your buttocks and lift up onto
your elbows to arch the back. Tuck your
chin in, then wriggle your shoulders
down as close to the buttocks as possible
to arch the spine.

2 **Exhale** Bring your feet flat to the floor just in front of your hips. Keep your feet parallel. Activate the abdominal and root locks in preparation for lifting.

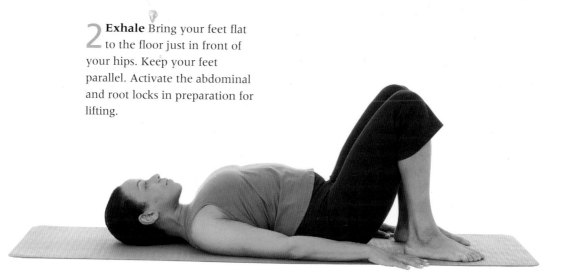

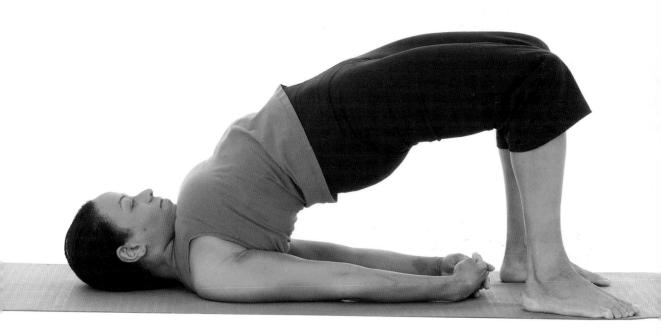

3 **Inhale** Keeping your hands tucked under your buttocks, lift your pelvis only off the floor. Once you are in position you may lace your fingers together and straighten your arms to achieve a higher lift. Hold the posture for five breaths in and out.

Exhale Lower to the floor. If you wish, repeat steps 1–3 for a total of three sets of five breaths each. Alternatively, try the full posture (see page 114).

Coming out

• **Exhale** After the final exhalation, come down and sit up with legs extended straight, ready for the counterpose.

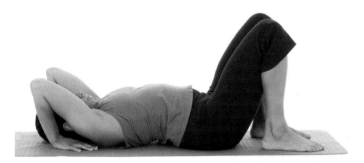

Full posture

• Bring your hands onto the floor at either side of your head, fingers pointing toward your shoulders. Activate the root and abdominal locks.

• **Inhale** Lift your pelvis and immediately push down with your hands and feet to lift up into the back bend. Hold the posture for five breaths in and out.

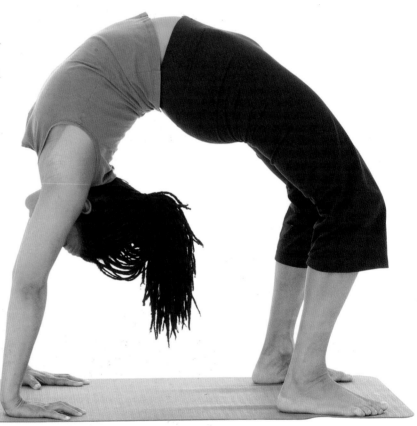

Repeating the pose

• **Exhale** Come down onto the top of your head. Adjust your hands: if you can, take them nearer your feet.
• **Inhale** Lift up again into the back bend.
• **Exhale** Lower and repeat three times in total, holding for five breaths each time.

Coming out

• **Exhale** After the final exhalation, come down and sit up with legs extended straight, ready for the counterpose.

Seated Forward Bend
(Paschimottanasana)

1 Inhale Grasp hold of the outside of your feet. If you are flexible enough, wrap your hands around your feet and hold onto one wrist. Lengthen your spine.

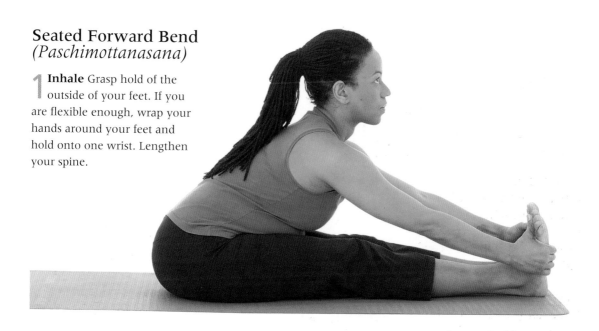

2 Exhale Fold forward over your legs, working your chin toward your shins. Look toward your toes and hold the posture for 10 breaths in and out.

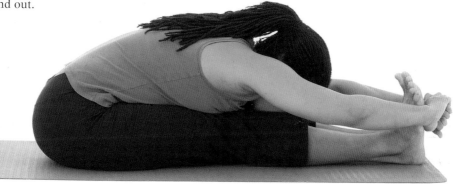

Coming out

• **Inhale** Arching your back, look up, maintaining the grip on your feet.

• **Exhale** Release your hands and come back to sitting.

• **Inhale** Do your Vinyasa.

Modified Shoulder Stand Sequence

Salamba Sarvangasana Before practising the postures in this lesson you must have completed all lessons up to and including Lesson 11. Take your time with this lesson, working toward the full variations of each posture in lesson 13 (see pages 120–127). When you can get your feet to the floor in Plough Posture you are ready to start the next lesson.

Benefits

Strengthens the nervous system and stimulates the thyroid and parathyroid, regulating metabolism. Aids the lymphatic system. Relieves symptoms of menopause.

Contraindications

Not suitable for those with heart problems, high blood pressure, detached retina or ear infections. Do not practise during menstruation.

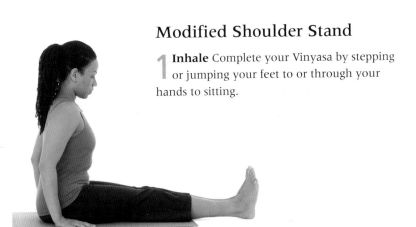

Modified Shoulder Stand

1 **Inhale** Complete your Vinyasa by stepping or jumping your feet to or through your hands to sitting.

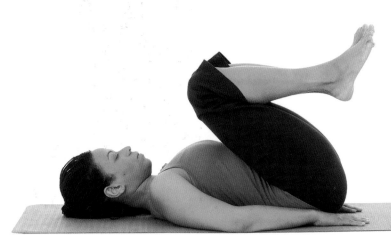

2 **Exhale** Lie down. Bend your knees toward your chest and tuck your thumbs beneath your buttocks.

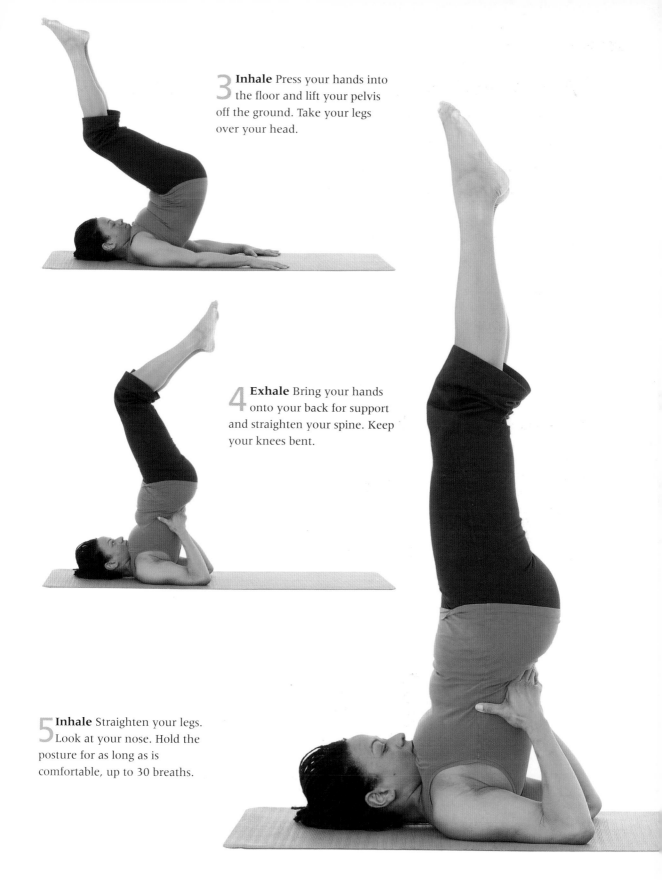

3 Inhale Press your hands into the floor and lift your pelvis off the ground. Take your legs over your head.

4 Exhale Bring your hands onto your back for support and straighten your spine. Keep your knees bent.

5 Inhale Straighten your legs. Look at your nose. Hold the posture for as long as is comfortable, up to 30 breaths.

Modified Plough Posture (*Halasana*)

1 **Exhale** Lower your legs over your head, keeping your hands in position to support your back unless you can bring your feet comfortably to the floor. If you can get your feet to the floor with your legs straight, then you are ready to try Lesson 13. Look at your nose. Hold the posture for up to 15 breaths.

Modified Ear Squeeze Posture (*Karnapidasana*)

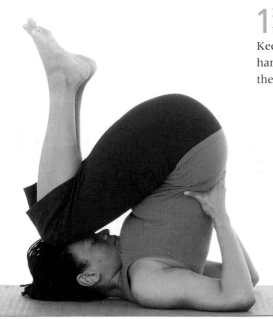

1 **Exhale** Bend your knees. Bring them to rest on your forehead. Keep your back supported by your hands. Looking at your nose, hold the posture for 10 breaths.

Coming out

• **Inhale** Straighten your legs and bring your arms to the floor, palms down.

• **Exhale** Lower your body to the floor until you are lying flat on your back. Tuck your thumbs beneath your buttocks, ready for the next modified posture.

Modified Leg Extension *(Uttanapadasana)*

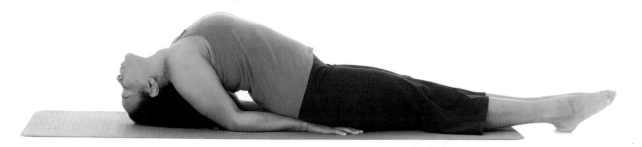

1 **Inhale** Lift up onto your elbows, lifting your back and head away from the ground. Arch your back and place the top of your head on the floor.

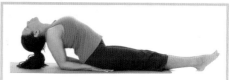

Step 1 – Working with stiffness
If you feel any neck pain in this posture, keep your head lifted off the ground.

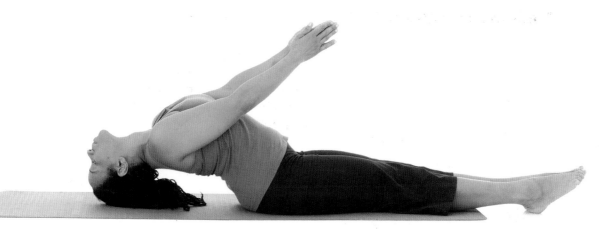

2 **Exhale** Release your hands from beneath your buttocks, and bring them up into Prayer Position above your chest, arms straight, pointing up at a 45-degree angle. Look at your nose. Hold the posture for five breaths in and out.

Coming out
• **Exhale** Release your arms and head.
• **Inhale** Hug your knees to your chest.
• **Exhale** Rock backward.
• **Inhale** Rock up to sitting and do your Vinyasa.

Full Shoulder Stand Sequence

Salamba Sarvangasana Before practising the postures in this section you must have completed all lessons up to Lesson 12. Once you are competent in Shoulder Stand, you may skip Lesson 12 and move straight from Lesson 11 to Lesson 13. After finishing the sequence, move on to the next lesson if you are ready or finish your practice with Lesson 15 (see pages 134–39).

Benefits

Strengthens the nervous system and stimulates the thyroid and parathyroid, regulating metabolism. Aids the lymphatic system. Relieves symptoms of menopause.

Contraindications

Not suitable for those with heart problems, high blood pressure, detached retina or ear infections. Do not practise during menstruation.

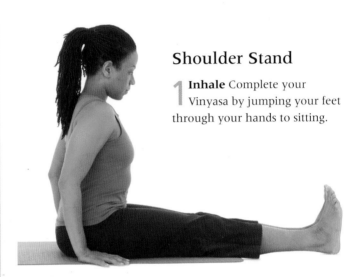

Shoulder Stand

1 Inhale Complete your Vinyasa by jumping your feet through your hands to sitting.

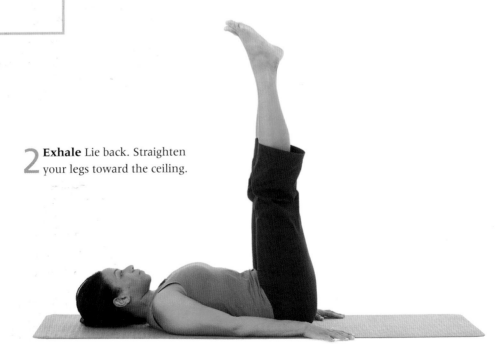

2 Exhale Lie back. Straighten your legs toward the ceiling.

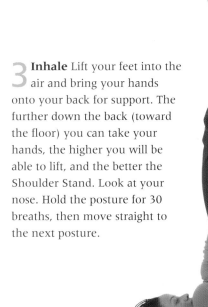

3 **Inhale** Lift your feet into the air and bring your hands onto your back for support. The further down the back (toward the floor) you can take your hands, the higher you will be able to lift, and the better the Shoulder Stand. Look at your nose. Hold the posture for 30 breaths, then move straight to the next posture.

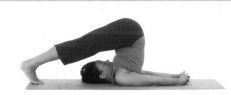

Step 3 – Perfecting the pose

It is far easier to lift into Shoulder Stand if you exhale into Plough Posture, lace your fingers, extend your arms and wriggle from side to side to lift high onto the shoulders. Keep your elbows in line, then bring your hands to your back and lift up into Shoulder Stand. There should be no strain or pressure in the neck. Keep the weight in your shoulders and arms.

Plough Posture
(Halasana)

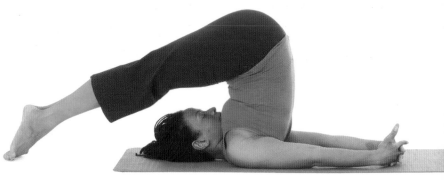

1 **Exhale** Folding from the hips, lace your hands and lower your feet to the floor behind your head. Interlace your fingers and straighten your arms. Keep your legs straight. If you can, point your toes. Look at your nose. Hold the posture for 15 breaths, then move straight to the next posture.

Ear Squeeze Posture
(Karnapidasana)

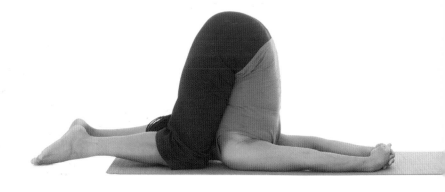

1 **Exhale** Bend your knees and bring them to the floor on either side of your head. Squeeze your ears with your knees. Keep your feet together. Look at your nose. Hold the posture for 10 breaths, then move straight to the next posture.

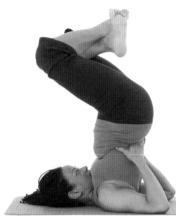

Face-up Lotus Posture
(Urdhva Padmasana)

1 **Inhale** Bring your hands back onto your back and lift up into Shoulder Stand.
Exhale Bend your knees and cross your ankles.

2 **Inhale** Take your hands to your knees. Press with your hands and straighten your arms completely, pushing your knees up. Look at your nose. Hold the posture for five breaths, then move straight to the next posture.

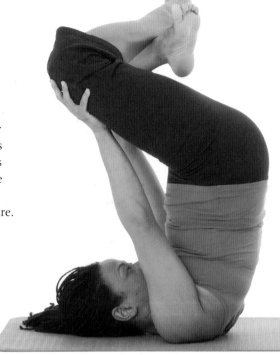

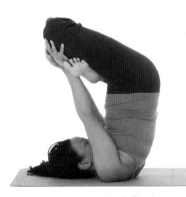

Full posture
• **Exhale** Bring your legs into Lotus Position, right leg first. Rest your knees on your hands.
• **Inhale** Take your hands to your knees and straighten arms.

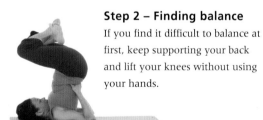

Step 2 – Finding balance
If you find it difficult to balance at first, keep supporting your back and lift your knees without using your hands.

Fetus Posture
(Pindasana)

1 **Exhale** Lower your knees to your ears, wrap your arms around your legs and hold your feet. Look at your nose. Hold the posture for five breaths in and out, then move straight to the next posture.

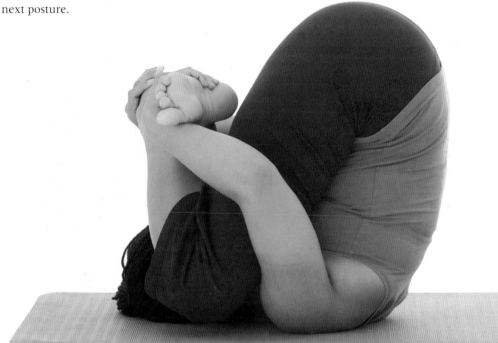

Full posture
• Still in Lotus Position, lower your knees to your ears, wrap your arms around your legs and bind your hands.

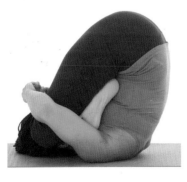

Coming out
• **Inhale** Release your arms to the floor, palms facing downward for support.
• **Exhale** Roll down with control, bringing your bottom to the floor as you maintain the cross-legged position.

Fish Posture
(Matsayasana)

1 Inhale Once your bottom reaches the floor, tuck your thumbs beneath your buttocks and lift onto your elbows. Arch your back and lower the top of your head to the floor.

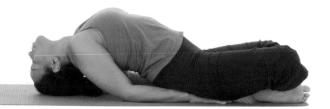

2 Exhale Take your hands beneath your legs and, if you can, hold your feet. Straightening your arms, push your chest out between them. Look at your third eye. Hold the posture for five breaths, then move straight to the next posture.

Full posture
• **Exhale** Remaining in Lotus Position, roll down.
• **Inhale** Lift onto your elbows, arch back and lower your head to the floor.
• **Exhale** Hold your feet and straighten your arms.

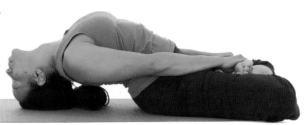

Leg Extension
(Uttanapadasana)

1 Inhale Release your legs
from the cross-legged or Lotus
Position, keeping your back
arched and the top of your head
on the floor. Lift your legs from
the floor at a 45-degree angle.

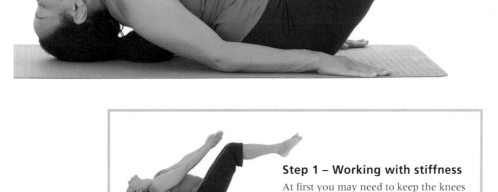

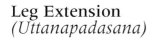

Step 1 – Working with stiffness

At first you may need to keep the knees
bent in this posture.

Full posture

• **Inhale** Bring your hands into
Prayer Position above the body,
arms straight, pointing up at a
45-degree angle. Look at your
nose. Hold the posture for five
breaths in and out.

• **Exhale** Release the posture
and lie flat on your back.

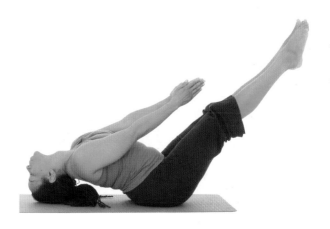

Wheel Posture *(Chakrasana)*

Only attempt this move if you are comfortable in all the Shoulder Stand variations. If you prefer, rock to sitting, as at the end of the modified sequence in Lesson 12 (see page 119).

1 **Inhale** Bend your knees toward your chest.

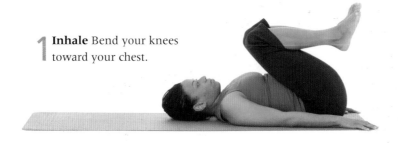

2 **Exhale** Place your hands on the floor on either side of your head.

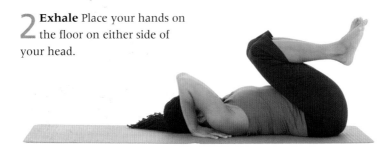

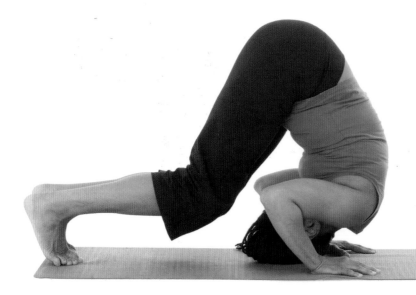

3 **Inhale** Swing your hips up into the air, bringing your knees over your head. As you do so, press with your hands and push your feet up and back.

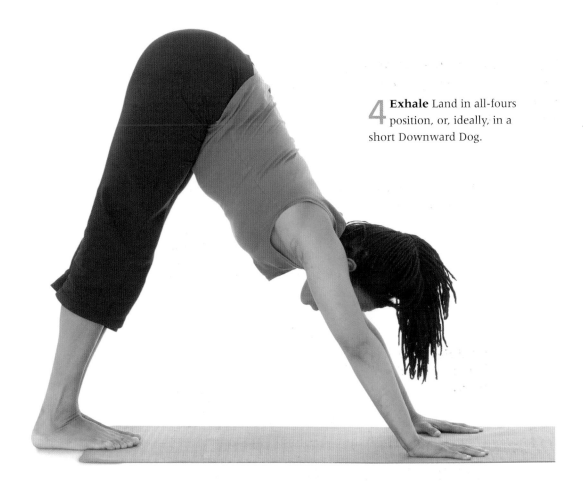

4 **Exhale** Land in all-fours position, or, ideally, in a short Downward Dog.

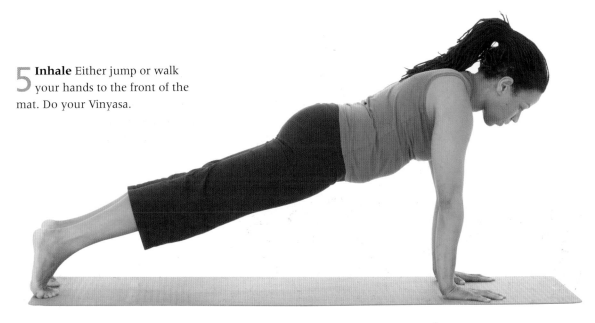

5 **Inhale** Either jump or walk your hands to the front of the mat. Do your Vinyasa.

Modified Head Stand

Sirsasana Before practising the postures in this section you must have completed all lessons up to and including Lesson 13. To learn Head Stand, start by using a wall. Once you can balance securely, you are ready to practise the Head Stand sequence away from the wall.

Benefits

Boosts the lymphatic system and is said to stimulate the brain and pituitary gland. All inversions are considered anti-ageing.

Contraindications

Not suitable for those with heart problems, high blood pressure, detached retina or ear infections. Do not practise during menstruation. Practise with care.

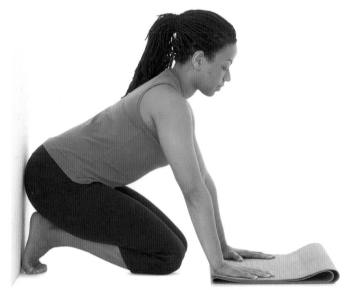

1 Pick up your mat, find a clear wall and kneel with your back to the wall, the balls of your feet touching the skirting board. Fold your mat once or twice and put it down directly in front of your knees.

2 To set the hand position, grasp your elbows and place them on the floor 10–15 cm (4–6 in) in front of your knees (any further forward and the posture won't work). Maintaining the elbow position, release your hands and interlace your fingers. Make a straight line from elbows to knuckles, wrists touching the floor. Don't stick your wrists out.

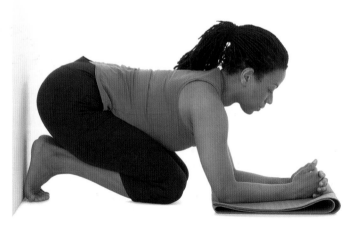

Step 2 – Positioning the hands

Most people find it easier to balance if the hands are cupped and the head is supported by the base of the thumbs. If this position doesn't work for you, you may need to open your hands and press your palms onto the back of your head.

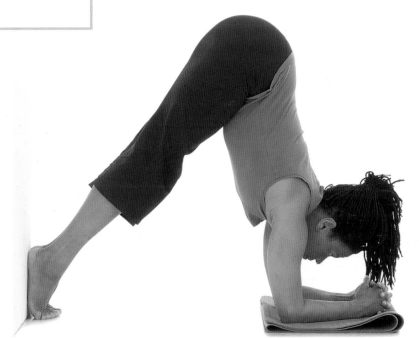

3 **Inhale** Straighten your legs and lift your hips. Notice the weight in your arms. This is what holds you up in the posture. Make this your Head Stand practice until you are ready to put weight on your head.

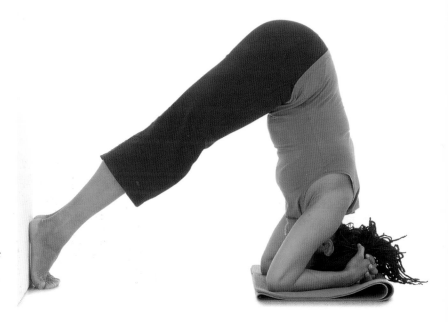

4 **Exhale** Place your head on the floor between your wrists, with the back of your head either pressing on the base of the thumbs or into the palms. Make sure the part of your head touching the floor is between the hairline (or where it once was) and the crown of your head.

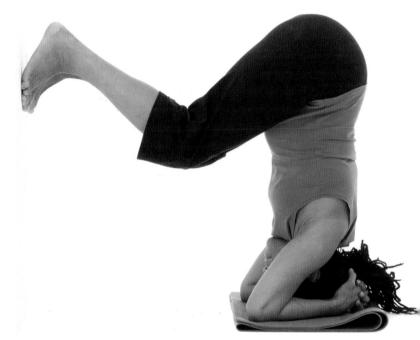

5 **Inhale** Step your feet onto the wall, level with your hips (no higher). Keep your knees bent until you are sure your feet are in the right position.

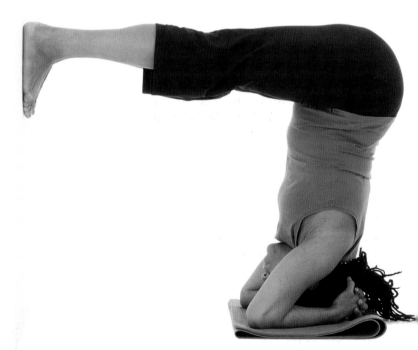

6 **Exhale** Straighten your legs to take your hips directly over your shoulders. Press your chest toward the wall, open your shoulders and lift up through your sitting bones. Hold this posture for 20 breaths, or move on and attempt to balance.

Balancing

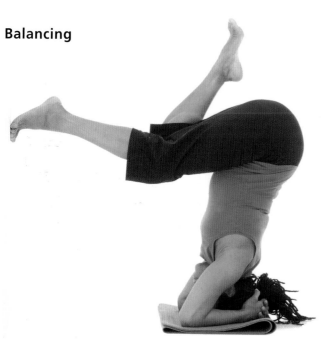

• **Keep breathing regularly** Point your toes so your hips move further into the room. When your body feels light, bend one knee at a time to come into a bent-legged Head Stand.

• **Inhale** In this position work on straightening your legs. Alternatively, lift your legs straight up into Head Stand, taking care to adjust the hips back to centre as you bring your legs up. Don't kick. Remember to breathe and use your bandhas.

Coming out

• **Exhale** Lower your feet to the floor and kneel. Keep your hands where they are or rest your arms on either side of your body. This is Child Posture. Relax for 10 breaths, then do your Vinyasa before proceeding to breathing and relaxation.

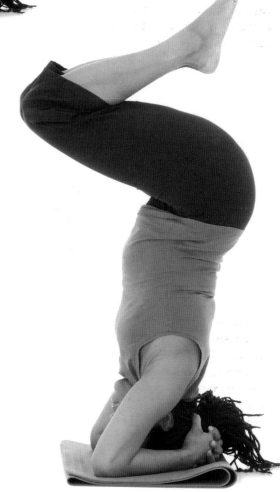

Head Stand

Sirsasana Do not attempt this posture until you are fully confident coming into Head Stand with the support of the wall. After finishing the posture, complete your practice with Lesson 15 (see pages 134–39).

Benefits

Boosts the lymphatic system and is said to stimulate the brain and pituitary gland. All inversions are considered anti-ageing.

Contraindications

Not suitable for those with heart problems, high blood pressure, detached retina or ear infections. Do not practise during menstruation. Practise with care.

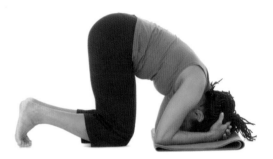

1 Exhale After Downward Dog, kneel and set your hand and head position.

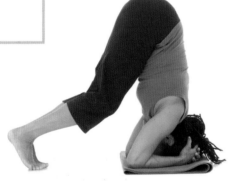

2 Inhale Lift your bottom and walk your feet towards your head until your feet lift off the floor. Don't kick!

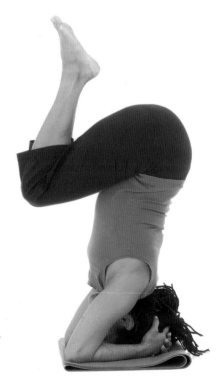

3 Exhale Once you are balancing with your knees bent, straighten your back. Stay here and breathe until you feel ready to go further.

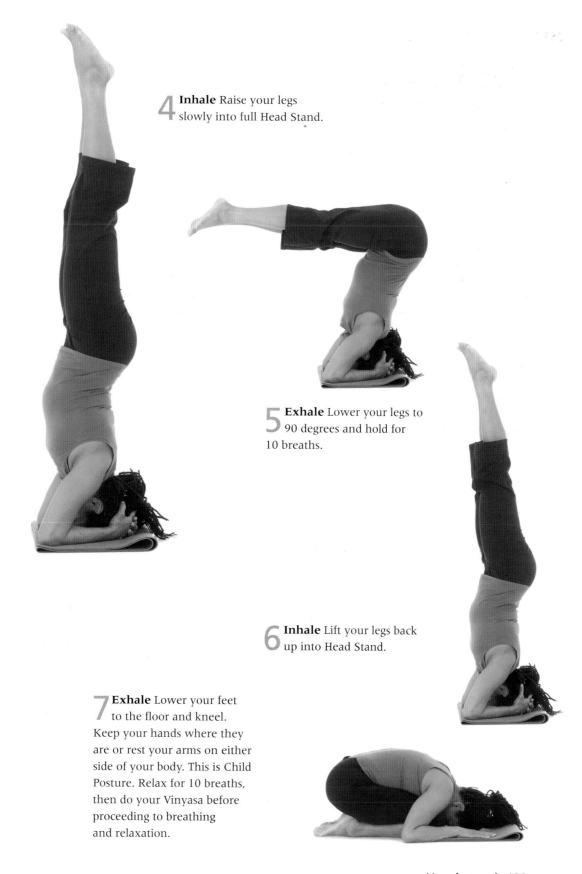

4 Inhale Raise your legs slowly into full Head Stand.

5 Exhale Lower your legs to 90 degrees and hold for 10 breaths.

6 Inhale Lift your legs back up into Head Stand.

7 Exhale Lower your feet to the floor and kneel. Keep your hands where they are or rest your arms on either side of your body. This is Child Posture. Relax for 10 breaths, then do your Vinyasa before proceeding to breathing and relaxation.

Breathing Sequence

Pranayama Use this set of postures at the end of your daily practice. Here the emphasis is on slowing and deepening the breath, while maintaining the Ujjayi sound. If you have just finished Lessons 1–4, sit down on your mat. If you have just completed Lesson 5, you will be sitting already. Following any of the other lessons, remember to do a Vinyasa between your last posture and the breathing sequence.

Benefits

Ujjayi breathing takes pressure into the throat allowing the nasal passages to clear completely for deeper breathing. It also balances the breath between nostrils, thought to improve the balance of active and passive elements in the body, allowing you to be both dynamic and relaxed during practice.

Contraindications

Very rarely can cause dizziness at first. If so, slow down until your body becomes used to deeper breathing.

Breathing Sequence in Easy Posture

1 Inhale Sit down on your mat.
Exhale Bring your right heel in front of your groin, then your left heel in front of your right ankle, taking your knees out to the side. This is Easy Posture (*Siddasana*).

Step 1 – Working with stiffness

If you cannot do Easy Posture, bring your legs to a cross-legged position. If this, too, is uncomfortable, place a book or cushion beneath your bottom when you start sitting to release the hips and lower back.

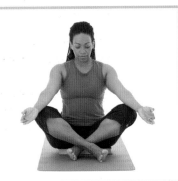

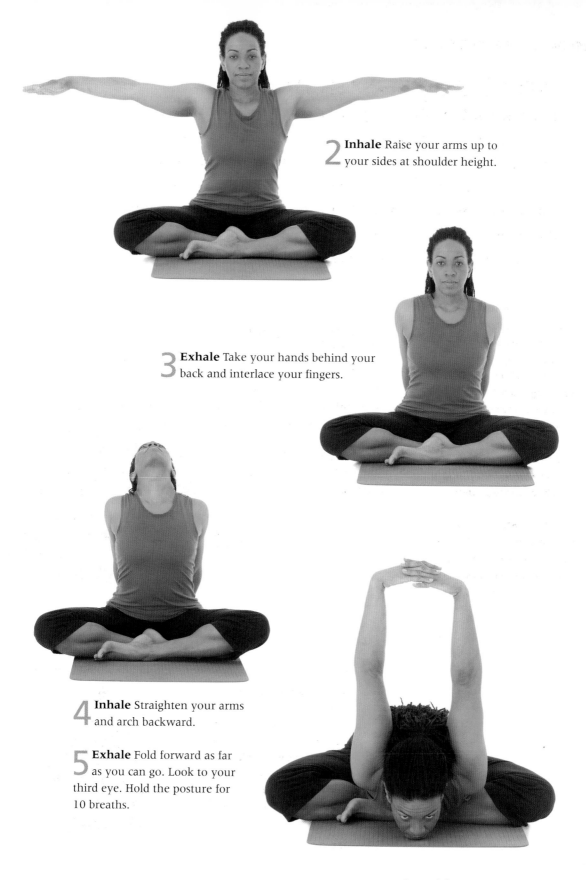

2 Inhale Raise your arms up to your sides at shoulder height.

3 Exhale Take your hands behind your back and interlace your fingers.

4 Inhale Straighten your arms and arch backward.

5 Exhale Fold forward as far as you can go. Look to your third eye. Hold the posture for 10 breaths.

Full Posture Bound Lotus Position (*Baddha Padmasana*)

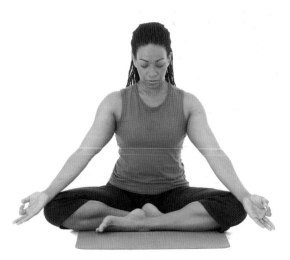

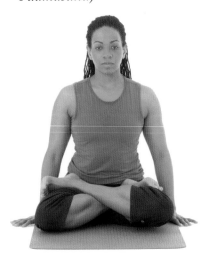

6 Inhale Sit up and release your hands. **Exhale** Bring the tips of your index fingers and thumbs together and rest the backs of your wrists on your knees. Look at your nose. Hold the posture for 20 breaths.

1 Inhale Bring your legs into full Lotus Position, right leg first, left foot on top.

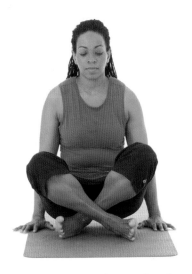

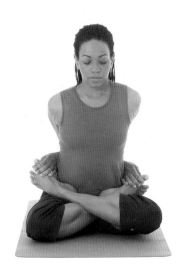

7 Exhale Raise your knees, then lean forward to bring your hands to the floor in front of your hips. **Inhale** Lift yourself off the ground, bottom first. Aim, eventually, to take your feet off the ground. Look at your nose. Hold the posture for 10 breaths. This is called *Uth Pluthi*.

2 Exhale Take your hands behind your back (left arm first) to bind your feet. **Inhale** Sit up and arch backward.

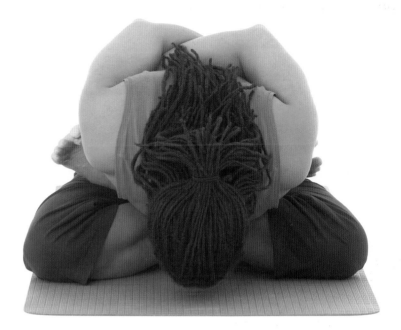

3 Exhale Fold forward for 10 breaths.

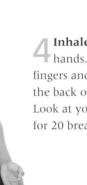

4 Inhale Sit up and release your hands. **Exhale** Bring your index fingers and thumbs together and rest the back of the wrists on your knees. Look at your nose. Hold the posture for 20 breaths.

Step 2 – Perfecting the pose

If you find it difficult to bind both hands, bind the left hand first. Release the left hand and use it to push your right elbow until you have bound the right foot, then rebind on the left. Keep folding forward while you try to bind.

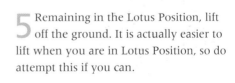

5 Remaining in the Lotus Position, lift off the ground. It is actually easier to lift when you are in Lotus Position, so do attempt this if you can.

Coming out

• **Exhale** Sit back on your mat.
• You may like to finish the breathing practice with an affirmation or prayer.

Relaxation

Savasana You should allow at least 10 minutes to rest in Savasana after a yoga session. Never skip relaxation! If you have practised up to Lesson 5, just lie down on your mat. If you are more advanced, do a Vinyasa, then lie down. Make sure you are warm enough during relaxation. The body cools quickly when motionless; you might like to cover yourself with a blanket.

Benefits

Allows the body to rest and heal and the mind to process what has been learned during the practice.

Contraindications

People with lower back pain may prefer to lie with knees bent, supported by a bolster or rolled-up blanket. Do not place a cushion beneath the head, which encourages incorrect alignment of the neck.

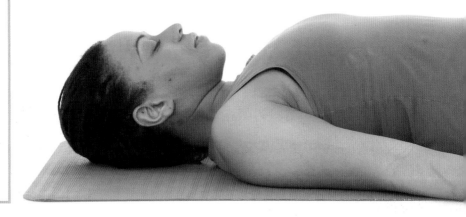

1 Lie on your back with your legs wider than hip distance apart and your arms out to the sides. Take a few deep breaths and sigh to release any tension in your body. You may want to shake your arms and legs, and move your head to make sure you have established a comfortable position. With eyes closed (use an eye mask if you find it helpful), breathe softly and naturally, allowing yourself to relax completely. Congratulate yourself! You have now completed your practice.

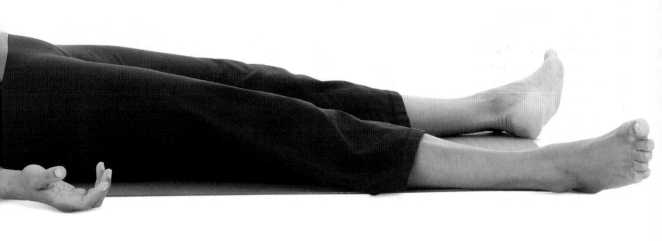

Quick reference chart

Photocopy this chart and stick it to a wall in front of you to remind you of the order of postures. It is best to cover all but the most recently learned postures and to rely on your memory to take you through the practice.

SUN SALUTATION A (LESSON 1)

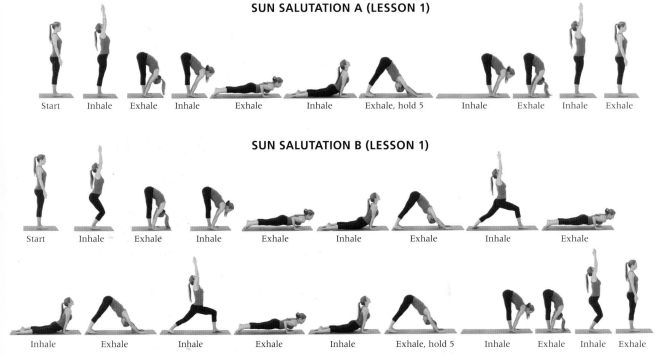

Start   Inhale   Exhale   Inhale   Exhale   Inhale   Exhale, hold 5   Inhale   Exhale   Inhale   Exhale

SUN SALUTATION B (LESSON 1)

Start   Inhale   Exhale   Inhale   Exhale   Inhale   Exhale   Inhale   Exhale

Inhale   Exhale   Inhale   Exhale   Inhale   Exhale, hold 5   Inhale   Exhale   Inhale   Exhale

STANDING POSES (LESSONS 2–4)

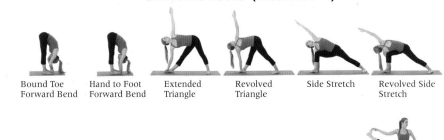

Bound Toe Forward Bend   Hand to Foot Forward Bend   Extended Triangle   Revolved Triangle   Side Stretch   Revolved Side Stretch

Wide-legged Forward Bend A   Wide-legged Forward Bend B   Wide-legged Forward Bend C   Wide-legged Forward Bend D   Lateral Forward Bend   Extended Leg Balance   Standing Half-bound Lotus Forward Bend

WARRIOR SEQUENCE (LESSON 5)

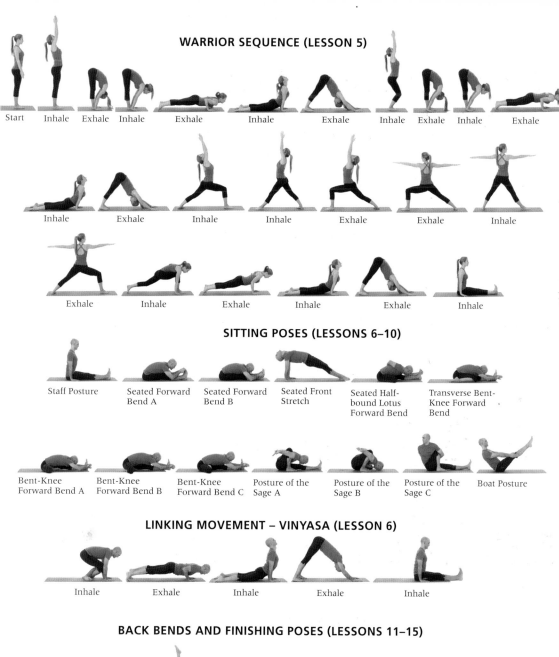

Start Inhale Exhale Inhale Exhale Inhale Exhale Inhale Exhale Inhale Exhale

Inhale Exhale Inhale Inhale Exhale Exhale Inhale

Exhale Inhale Exhale Inhale Exhale Inhale

SITTING POSES (LESSONS 6–10)

Staff Posture Seated Forward Bend A Seated Forward Bend B Seated Front Stretch Seated Half-bound Lotus Forward Bend Transverse Bent-Knee Forward Bend

Bent-Knee Forward Bend A Bent-Knee Forward Bend B Bent-Knee Forward Bend C Posture of the Sage A Posture of the Sage B Posture of the Sage C Boat Posture

LINKING MOVEMENT – VINYASA (LESSON 6)

Inhale Exhale Inhale Exhale Inhale

BACK BENDS AND FINISHING POSES (LESSONS 11–15)

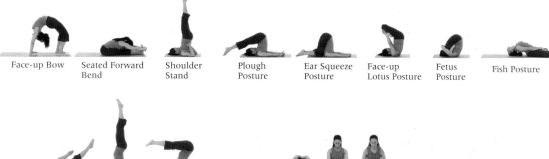

Face-up Bow Seated Forward Bend Shoulder Stand Plough Posture Ear Squeeze Posture Face-up Lotus Posture Fetus Posture Fish Posture

Leg Extension Head Stand Head Stand Variation Child Posture Breathing Sequence Relaxation

Index

A

anjusta ma dyai (thumbs gaze) 17
Ardha Baddha Padma Paschimottanasana (Seated Half-bound Lotus Forward Bend) 92–3
Ardha Baddha Padmottanasana (Standing Half-bound Lotus Forward Bend) 72–3
Ashtanga Vinyasa Yoga 6–7

B

back bending 112–15
back pain 9
Baddha Padmasana (Full Posture Bound Lotus Position) 136–7
bandha (locks) 17, 19
beginning inversions 116–19
Bent-Knee Forward Bends 96–101
Boat Posture 108–9
body locks 17, 19
Bound Toe Forward Bend 46–7
breathing 16–21
Breathing Sequence 134–7
broomadhya (third eye gaze) 17

C

Chakrasana (Wheel Posture) 126–7
Child Posture 133

D

dizziness 9
Downward Dog Posture
    Linking Movement 89
    Sun Salutations 25, 30, 36, 38, 41, 43, 44
    Warrior Sequence 76, 78, 81

Wheel Posture 127
dristi (gaze point) 17

E

Ear Squeeze Posture 118, 121
Easy Posture 134–6
Extended Leg Balance 70–1
Extended Triangle 50–1

F

Face-up Bow 112–14
Face-up Lotus Posture 122
Fetus Posture 123
finishing poses 110–39
Fish Posture 124
Forward Bends
    Bent-Knee 96–101
    Bound Toe 46–7
    Hand to Foot 48–9
    Lateral 66–7
    Seated 84–7, 115
    Seated Half-bound Lotus 92–3
    Standing 62–7
    Standing Half-bound Lotus 72–3
    Transverse Bent-Knee 94–5
    Wide-legged 58–65
foundation postures 48–61
Front Stretch, Seated 90–1
Full Posture Bound Lotus Position 136–7
Full Shoulder Stand Sequence 120–1

G

gaze points 17

H

Halasana (Plough Posture) 118, 121
Half-lotus Position 92
hamstring injury 9
hand gaze 17
Hand to Foot Forward Bend 48–9
hastagrai (hand gaze) 17
Head Stand 128–33
Hip Rotators 92–5

I

illness 8
injury 8, 9
inversions, beginning 116–19

J

Janu Sirsasana (Bent-Knee Forward Bends) 96–101

K

Karnapidasana (Ear Squeeze Posture) 118, 121
knee pain 9

L

Lateral Forward Bend 66–7
Leg Balances 68–73
    Utthita Hasta Padangusthasana 68–71
Leg Extension 119, 125
Linking Movement 88–9
locks 17, 19
Lotus Position
    Face-up Posture 122
    Fetus Posture 123
    Full Posture Bound 136–7
    Half- 92
    Posture of the Sage 104
lower back pain 9

M

Marichyasana (Posture of the Sage) 102–7
mats 10
Matsayasana (Fish Posture) 124
menstruation 8
Modified Ear Squeeze Posture 118
Modified Head Stand 128–31
Modified Leg Balance 68–9
Modified Leg Extension 119
Modified Plough Posture 118
Modified Shoulder Stand Sequence 116–17
moving with breath 20–1
Mula Bandha (root lock) 17, 19

N

nabi chakra (navel gaze) 17
nasagrai (nose gaze) 17
Navasana (Boat Posture) 108–9
navel gaze 17
neck pain 9
Neutral Position 20
nose gaze 17

P

Padahastasana (Hand to Foot Forward Bend) 48–9
Padangusthasana (Bound Toe Forward Bend) 46–7
padhayoragrai (toes gaze) 17
pain 9
Parivrtta Parsvakonasana (Revolved Side Stretch) 56–7
Parivrtta Trikonasana (Revolved Triangle) 52–3
parsva (sideways gaze) 17
Parsvottanasana (Lateral Forward Bend) 66–7
partners 11
Paschimottanasana (Seated Forward Bend) 84–7, 115
Patanjali 7
Pattabhi Jois, Sri K 6, 7, 12
Pindasana (Fetus Posture) 123
Plough Posture 118, 121
Posture of the Sage 102–7
practising safely 8–9
Pranayama (Breathing Sequence) 134–7
Prasarita Padottanasana (Wide-legged Forward Bends) 58–65
Prayer Position 28
pregnancy 8
Primary Series 7, 12
problems 9
Purvattanasana (Seated Front Stretch) 90–1

R

Rangaswami, Sharath 7
reference chart 140–1

Relaxation 138
Revolved Side Stretch 56–7
Revolved Triangle 52–3
root lock 17, 19

S

safe practise 8–9
Sage Postures 102–7
Salamba Sarvangasana (Shoulder Stand Sequence) 116–17, 120–1
Samasthitih (Neutral Position) 20
Savasana (Relaxation) 138
Seat of Power (*Utkatasana*) 76
Seated Forward Bend 84–7, 115
Seated Front Stretch 90–1
Seated Half-bound Lotus Forward Bend 92–3
shoulder pain 9
Shoulder Stand Sequence 116–17, 120–7
  Salamba Sarvangasana 116–17, 120–1
Siddasana (Easy Posture) 134–6
Side Stretch 54–5
sideways gaze 17
Sirsasana (Head Stand) 128–33
sitting basics 84–91
sitting poses 82–109
Staff Posture 84–6
Standing Forward Bends 62–7
Standing Half-bound Lotus Forward Bend 72–3
standing poses 14–81
Sun Salutations 12, 22–45
Surya Namaskara (Sun Salutations) 12, 22–45

T

third eye gaze 17
thumbs gaze 17
Tiriangmukhaikapada Paschimottanasana (Transverse Bent-Knee Forward Bend) 94–5

toes gaze 17
Transverse Bent-Knee Forward Bend 94–5
Triangle
  Extended 50–1
  Revolved 52–3

U

Uddiyana Bandha (upward flying seal) 17, 19
Ujjayi breathing (victorious breathing) 16, 18
Upward Dog Posture
  Linking Movement 89
  Sun Salutations 25, 29, 33, 36, 38, 41, 42, 44
  Warrior Sequence 75, 77, 81
upward flying seal 17, 19
upward gaze 17
urdhva (upward gaze) 17
Urdhva Dhanurasana (Face-up Bow) 112–14
Urdhva Padmasana (Face-up Lotus Posture) 122
Utkatasana (Seat of Power) 76
Virabhadrasana (Warrior Sequence) 74–81
Uttanapadasana (Leg Extension) 119, 125
Utthita Hasta Padangusthasana (Leg Balance) 68–71
Utthita Parsvakonasana (Side Stretch) 54–5
Utthita Trikonasana (Extended Triangle) 50–1

V

victorious breathing 16, 18
Vinyasa 7, 16–17
  Linking Movement 88–9

W

Warrior Sequence 74–81
Wheel Posture 126–7
Wide-legged Forward Bends 58–65
wrists 9

Acknowledgements

I would like to thank my wonderful teachers,
too numerous to mention, but including Sri K
Pattabhi Jois, Sharath Rangaswami, Derek
Ireland, Radha Warrell, John Scott, and all of
my dear students.

Executive Editor   Jo Godfreywood
Managing Editor   Clare Churly
Executive Art Editor   Leigh Jones
Designer   Bridget Morley
Photographer   Mike Good
Production Controller   Simone Nauerth